In 2006, over 74 percent of American women were breast-feeding newborns. But only 43 percent were still nursing their babies by the sixth month, and this dropped to less than 23 percent by their first birthday. Based on the latest research and the American Academy of Pediatrics' breastfeeding policy statement, this essential handbook answers new mothers' most common questions about breastfeeding, including:

- How will I know if my baby is getting enough milk?
- What kind of diet is best while breastfeeding?
- Is my baby latched on properly?
- Will I be able to breastfeed once I return to work?
- How can I keep my partner involved while I breastfeed?
- How can I get friends and family to support this important decision?
- How do I breastfeed a teething toddler?
- At what age do I wean my child—and how?
- Can I still breastfeed after breast surgery?
- Will taking aspirin or other medications adversely affect my breastfeeding baby?

. . . and much more, to help you and your baby get the healthiest possible start. The benefits will last a lifetime.

AMERICAN ACADEMY OF PEDIATRICS

New MOTHER'S GUIDE *to* BREASTFEEDING

Second Edition

Joan Younger Meek,
M.D., M.S., R.D., FAAP, IBCLC,
Editor in Chief

with Winnie Yu

BANTAM BOOKS TRADE PAPERBACKS
New York

2011 Bantam Books Trade Paperback Edition

Copyright © 2002, 2011 by the American Academy of Pediatrics

All rights reserved.

Published in the United States by Bantam Books, an imprint of
The Random House Publishing Group,
a division of Random House, Inc., New York.

BANTAM BOOKS and colophon are trademarks of Random House, Inc.

This work was originally published in different form in the United States
by Bantam Books, an imprint of The Random House Publishing Group,
a division of Random House, Inc., in 2002.

AAP ISBN 978-1-58110-459-2

The Library of Congress has cataloged the earlier edition as follows:

American Academy of Pediatrics new mother's guide to breastfeeding /
Joan Younger Meek, editor-in-chief, with Sherill Tippins.
p. cm.
Includes bibliographical references and index.
ISBN 0-553-38107-5
1. Breast feeding.   I. Title: New mother's guide to breastfeeding.
II. Meek, Joan Younger.   III. Tippins, Sherill.   IV. American Academy
of Pediatrics.
RJ216.A477 2002
649'.33—dc21   2002023885

Printed in the United States of America on acid-free paper

2 4 6 8 9 7 5 3 1

Book design by Donna Sinisgalli

Acknowledgments

Editor in Chief
Joan Younger Meek, M.D., M.S., R.D., FAAP, IBCLC

AAP Board of Directors Reviewer
Edward N. Bailey, M.D., FAAP

Reviewers/Contributors
Jatinder J. S. Bhatia, M.D., FAAP
Linda Sue Black, M.D., FAAP
Antoinette P. Eaton, M.D., FAAP
Lori Feldman-Winter, M.D., FAAP
Lawrence M. Gartner, M.D., FAAP
Nancy F. Krebs, M.D., FAAP
Susan Landers, M.D., FAAP
Ruth A. Lawrence, M.D., FAAP
Lawrence M. Noble, M.D., FAAP
Yvette Piovanetti, M.D., FAAP
Nancy Powers, M.D., FAAP
John Queenan, M.D., FACOG
Wendelin Slusser, M.D., FAAP
Kinga A. Szucs, M.D., IBCLC, FAAP
Laura R. Viehmann, M.D., FAAP

Additional Assistance
Lauren Barone, MPH
Linda Diamond
Heather Fitzpatrick, MPH
Shannan Martin

Writer
Winnie Yu
Sherrill Tippins (first edition)

Illustrator
Tony LeTourneau, Rolin Graphics, Inc.

Editors
Robin Michaelson (first edition)
Stacie Fine (first edition)

Dedication

This book is dedicated to all the people who recognize that children are our greatest inspiration in the present and our greatest hope for the future.

The American Academy of Pediatrics recognizes that breastfeeding is important for the optimal health and development of infants and children. This publication was developed in gratitude to those mothers and professionals who have preserved breastfeeding in our culture and in the hope that increasing numbers of women in present and future generations will experience this unique opportunity to both nourish and nurture their children. It is our desire that women who read this book will find encouragement to make the decision to breastfeed, help for the early breastfeeding days, practical solutions for breastfeeding challenges, resources to help meet their personal goals for breastfeeding, and support to continue breastfeeding for as long as they choose.

From Joan Younger Meek, editor in chief:
I extend my personal thanks to Sandy Thompson, whose mother-to-mother support in encouraging me to breastfeed my children ultimately changed my career path; to Katie, Rachel, and Joseph, for teaching me how to be a breastfeeding mother; to Joshua and Nicholas, for showing me the joys of being a grandmother; to Paul, for supporting my advocacy of breastfeeding; to Dr. Deborah Squire, for mentoring me in becoming a breastfeeding-supportive pediatrician; and to the families who have entrusted me with the care of their children in my practice of pediatrics.

Please Note

The information contained in this book is intended to complement, not substitute for, the advice of your child's pediatrician. Before starting any medical treatment or medical program, you should consult with your own pediatrician, who can discuss your individual needs and counsel you about symptoms and treatment. If you have any questions regarding how the information in this book applies to your child, speak with your child's pediatrician.

The information and advice in this book apply equally to children of both sexes (except where noted). To indicate this, we have chosen to alternate between masculine and feminine pronouns throughout the book.

Foreword

The American Academy of Pediatrics (AAP) welcomes you to the second edition of *New Mother's Guide to Breastfeeding*.

Breastfeeding can give your baby the best possible start in life. This book will help mothers and all who care for children understand the neurologic, psychologic, and immunologic benefits of human milk; prepare for breastfeeding before a baby is born; plan for the first feeding and bringing the baby home; understand the father's role in breastfeeding; continue breastfeeding if the mother returns to work; and so much more.

This book is unique because pediatricians who specialize in breastfeeding have extensively reviewed it. Under the direction of our editor in chief, the material in this book was developed with the assistance of numerous contributors from the American Academy of Pediatrics. Because medical information is constantly changing, every effort has been made to ensure that this book contains the most up-to-date findings. Readers may want to visit the official AAP website for parents at www.HealthyChildren.org to keep current on this and other subjects.

It is our hope that this book will become an invaluable resource and reference guide for parents. We are confident that parents and caregivers will find the book extremely helpful. We encourage its use in concert with the advice and counsel of our readers' pediatricians, who will provide individual guidance and assistance related to the health of children.

The AAP is an organization of sixty thousand primary care pediatricians, pediatric medical subspecialists, and pediatric surgical specialists dedicated to the health, safety, and well-being of infants, children, adolescents, and young adults. This subsequent edition of *New Mother's Guide to Breastfeeding* is part of the Academy's ongoing educational efforts to provide parents and caregivers with high-quality information on a broad spectrum of children's health issues.

Errol R. Alden, M.D., FAAP
Executive Director
American Academy of Pediatrics

Contents

AMERICAN ACADEMY OF PEDIATRICS

New MOTHER'S
GUIDE *to*
BREASTFEEDING

CHAPTER 1

Choosing to Breastfeed

Congratulations—you're pregnant! Chances are you're experiencing a flood of emotions and preparing for a new life with your baby. You are probably also pondering some decisions, both big and small. *Where will the baby sleep when she comes home from the hospital? Will I stay at my job? Who will watch my baby if I go back to work?*

Among the most important decisions you'll make is whether to breastfeed your new baby. The decision to breastfeed is intensely personal and one that has important ramifications for your baby's health as well as yours. But like most women, you probably have questions about what breastfeeding entails, exactly how to nurse your child, and whether breastfeeding will fit into your lifestyle, schedule, and circumstances. Breastfeeding has both long- and short-term benefits for both you and your infant, including preventing many illnesses. Ultimately, only you will be able to determine whether breastfeeding is right for you, but the information in this book is designed to help you make that decision.

DOES BREASTFEEDING MAKE SENSE FOR ME?

The act of breastfeeding—one of nature's most rewarding and beneficial processes—can sometimes seem intimidating when you face a host of other commitments and hear a great deal of conflicting advice. In the following chapters, you will find clear answers to

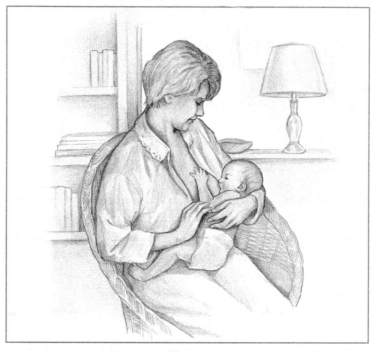

Breastfeeding ensures the healthiest start to an infant's life and provides important benefits for both mother and baby.

many of your questions, solutions to your problems, and information about the array of breastfeeding support services—hospital nurses, pediatricians, obstetricians, family physicians, lactation specialists, and breastfeeding support groups—that are in place to help mothers breastfeed their infants successfully.

Such efforts have been made because an enormous amount of research demonstrates how beneficial breastfeeding is for babies. We now know that nursing your child not only strengthens the quality of your relationship with her but also improves her health, enhances her brain development, and provides her with precisely the type of nourishment she needs at each critical stage of her development. The benefits of human milk so greatly exceed that of any alternative method of infant feeding, in fact, that health organizations around the globe have united to promote this natural source of nutritional and emotional sustenance for babies. The World Health Organization (WHO), for example, encourages women to breastfeed exclusively for six months (nothing but human milk) and to continue to breastfeed for at least two years to take advantage of human milk's ability to provide the best nutrition and protection against infection. Exclusive breastfeeding for six months has also been recommended by the American College of Obstetricians and Gynecologists, the American Academy of Family Physicians, the Academy of Breastfeeding Medicine, and the American Dietetic Association. The American Academy of Pedi-

---

Where We Stand

As the United States' foremost association of board-certified pediatricians, the American Academy of Pediatrics is committed to improving the health of all children. We recognize breastfeeding's role in creating the best possible health, developmental, and psychosocial outcomes for the infant. Therefore, we recommend breastfeeding as the sole source of nutrition for infants for at least four and preferably six months; breastfeeding in combination with complementary solid foods through at least twelve months; and continued breastfeeding thereafter for as long as mutually desired by mother and baby. While the ultimate decision to breastfeed is yours, it is our responsibility to provide you with complete, up-to-date information on the benefits and methods of breastfeeding to ensure that your feeding decision is a fully informed one. (For more information about the AAP's breastfeeding recommendations and policies, please log on to the AAP website for parents, www.HealthyChildren.org.)

atrics (AAP) recommends exclusive breastfeeding for a minimum of four but preferably six months of life. Exclusive breastfeeding means no water, formula, other liquids, or solids. Breastfeeding should then be continued for at least one year and thereafter as long as mutually desired by the mother and baby, with the appropriate introduction of complementary foods beginning around six months of age.

As you prepare for motherhood, you will want answers to all of your questions about breastfeeding. You will want to consider how it is possible to combine breastfeeding with work outside the home, how you can fully involve your partner in parenting a breastfed infant, and how to adjust if breastfeeding doesn't begin smoothly. You will need to understand how breastfeeding works so you can feel assured that certain behaviors are normal or recognize any difficulties. Finally, you will want to find knowledgeable breastfeeding support services in your area.

As pediatricians, we want to share all we know to help you reach your breastfeeding goals. With this guide, we will provide information, encouragement, and support as you learn this vital new skill. We will show you how many millions of women—working outside the home or not, married or not, first-time or experienced mothers—have provided the best for their babies through breastfeeding, and how you can too.

DID MY MOTHER BREASTFEED?

When you were an infant you may not have been breastfed, though your mother may have been and your grandmother was even more likely to have been breastfed. Breastfeeding, like many other aspects of nurturing children, has passed in and out of fashion according to parental and societal trends and the accumulation of reliable research.

Of course, few alternatives were available to mothers a century ago. In the early 1900s, the majority of American women breastfed their infants, and over half of the babies were still being breastfed beyond the first year of life. Mothers who could not or chose not to breastfeed or weaned early used a wet nurse, fed animal milk to their babies, or fed mixtures of flour, rice, and water called "pap." The newborns' chances of survival decreased significantly as a result. During the decades that followed, however, glass bottles and rubber nipples became more widely available and pasteurization and vitamin supplementation more commonplace. As a result, alternatives to breastfeeding became more practical and prevalent, though almost nothing was known about how these artificial infant feedings affected children's long-term health and development. During World War II, as more women worked outside the home, formula-feeding rose even more and continued to increase through the 1950s and 1960s. By 1966, only 18 percent of babies were being breastfed at the time they left the hospital, and this percentage dropped sharply soon after the babies arrived home. In the early 1970s in the United States, breastfeeding rates hit a record low.

At about this time, however, medical research began to uncover a wealth of information about the advantages of mother's milk for infant health and development. Scientists noted that formula-fed babies were more susceptible to diseases in the environment. They caught more colds, suffered from more ear infections, and experienced more allergies. Such findings, along with the mid-seventies movement toward a more natural childbirth and parenting experience, caused breastfeeding rates to climb again. In 1982, nearly 62 percent of newborns were nourished by their mother's milk after birth. By 2006, this number increased to almost 74 percent. Unfortunately, work conflicts and lack of support caused many mothers to give up nursing quite early, and this continues to be the case. Based upon the 2006 National Immunization Survey, only about 43 percent of American newborns were receiving any human milk by their sixth month, dropping to less than 23 percent by their first birthday. Only 33 percent were exclusively breastfed for the first three months of life. More than 25 percent of breastfed infants are given infant formula before they even leave the delivery hospital, and this figure is rising. Yet studies keep revealing the fascinating ways in which the content of human milk changes to suit the baby at every stage of development, continuing to provide precisely the developmental, psychological, and health benefits a baby needs through the first year and beyond.

Today, mothers are not forced to choose between only two alternatives—breastfeeding their babies or giving them formula. They may opt to breastfeed their babies directly; provide them with bottles of human milk that they have expressed and stored for later use; provide donated, processed human milk from a milk bank when their own milk production is insufficient or their milk cannot be used; or use commercially produced formula available in supermarkets and pharmacies as either a supplement to their own milk or a replacement for breastfeeding in the rare case that breastfeeding is not possible. The option you choose at any particular time will depend on your circumstances and you and your baby's needs. However, before you make your decision, you owe it to your baby to learn how breastfeeding benefits you both, and the advantages and disadvantages of each option. While the *best* outcomes for health and well-being are related to exclusive breastfeeding, alternatives can also provide benefits. Consider the support services (lactation specialists, breastfeeding support groups, and online information), efficient aids to breastfeeding (breast pumps, human milk storage containers), and increased social acceptance (more breastfeeding in public, maternity leave, private rooms provided at work for nursing mothers, "lactation workstations" at the workplace, and legislative support) now available to help you succeed. It is our hope that as you read about how breastfeeding benefits you and your baby and consider how nursing can be a part of your life, you will decide to breastfeed. After all, babies are not babies for very long. They deserve the healthiest start they can get.

WHY IS BREASTFEEDING SO GOOD FOR MY BABY?

Formula for babies has become such a pervasive part of our culture that many people assume it must be as good for babies as human milk. After all, formula is designed to contain many of the nutrients provided in human milk—and babies who are fed formula clearly grow adequately. Yet the fact remains that human milk and infant formula differ in a number of fundamental ways. Human milk is such a rich, nourishing mixture that scientists have yet to identify all of its elements, and no formula manufacturer has managed to duplicate it or will ever be able to fully replicate it. In addition, the act of breastfeeding, which involves nurturing and parenting behaviors, and specific hormonal responses for both mother and baby triggered by skin-to-skin contact, goes well beyond the analysis of the scientific ingredients of human milk.

∞ IMMUNOLOGIC BENEFITS

Human milk provides virtually all the protein, sugar, and fat your baby needs to be healthy, and it also contains many substances that benefit your baby's immune system, including antibodies, immune factors, enzymes, and white blood cells. These substances protect your baby against a wide variety of diseases and infections not only while he is breastfeeding but in some cases long after he has weaned. Formula cannot offer this protection.

If you develop a cold while breastfeeding, for example, you are likely to pass the cold germs on to your baby—but the antibodies your body produces to fight that cold also will be passed on through your milk. These antibodies will help your infant conquer the cold germs quickly and effectively and possibly avoid developing the cold altogether. This defense against illnesses significantly decreases the chances that your breastfeeding baby will suffer from ear infections, vomiting, diarrhea, pneumonia, urinary tract infections, or certain types of spinal meningitis. Infants under the age of one who breastfed exclusively for at least four months, for instance, were less likely to be hospitalized for a lower respiratory tract infection, such as croup, bronchiolitis, or pneumonia, than were their formula-fed counterparts. Even infants in group child care programs, who tend to catch more germs due to their close proximity, are less likely to become ill if they are breastfed or fed their mothers' milk in a bottle.

All humans have a very large number of bacteria that normally reside in their intestines. Some of the bacteria serve normal and healthy functions, and some can cause disease such as diarrhea. Human milk encourages the growth of healthy bacteria in the intestinal tract of the breastfed baby. It does this by promoting a generally healthy environment and, in part, through substances called prebiotics, which are found in human milk. Since human milk stimulates the growth of these "friendly" strains of bacteria, other bacteria such as *E. coli,* which are more likely to cause disease, are inhibited from growing, multiplying, and attaching to the lining of the intestine, where they can cause infection. It has been well established that formula-fed infants have much higher rates of diarrheal diseases which may require visits to the doctor or sometimes to the hospital for intravenous fluids.

Breastfeeding is recommended for many reasons. With regard to allergy prevention, there is some evidence that breastfeeding protects babies born to families with a history of allergies, compared to those babies who are fed either a standard cow's-milk-based formula or a soy formula. In these "at risk" families, breastfed babies generally had a lower risk of milk allergy, atopic dermatitis (commonly known as eczema), and wheezing early in life, if they were exclusively breastfed for at least four months. It is presumed that immune components in maternal milk provide protection against these allergic diseases. Although the long-term benefits of breastfeeding on allergies remains unclear and studies have not carefully evaluated the impact on families without a history of allergy, exclusive breastfeeding is recommended as the feeding of choice for all infants.

Transfer of the human milk antibodies and other immunologic substances may also explain why children who breastfeed for more than six months are less likely to develop childhood acute leukemia and lymphoma than those who receive formula. In addition, studies have demonstrated a 36 percent reduction (some studies show this reduction to be as high as 50 percent) in risk of sudden infant death syndrome (SIDS) among babies who breastfeed compared to those who did not, though the reasons for this are not fully understood. Recent research even indicates that breastfed infants are less likely to be obese in adolescence and adulthood. They are also less vulnerable to developing both type 1 and type 2 diabetes.

Health Benefits

Research has shown that babies who are breastfed reap numerous benefits. Compared to those who are breastfed, babies who are formula-fed have higher rates of the following:

- Ear infections
- Eczema, food allergies, and asthma
- Gastrointestinal infections that cause vomiting and diarrhea
- Pneumonia and other respiratory diseases
- Obesity in adolescence and adulthood
- Type 1 and type 2 diabetes
- Childhood leukemia and lymphoma
- Sudden infant death syndrome (SIDS)

Ip S, Chung M, Raman G, et al. *Breastfeeding and Maternal and Infant Health Outcomes in Developed Countries.* Evidence Report/Technology Assessment No. 153. Rockville, MD: Agency for Healthcare Research and Quality; 2007. AHRQ Publication No. 07-E007. www.ahrq.gov/downloads/pub/evidence/pdf/brfout/brfout.pdf. Accessed August 6, 2010.

∞   HUMAN MILK AND INFANT DEVELOPMENT

In addition to being able to help defend against threats in the environment, the composition of human milk adjusts over time to meet your child's needs at each stage of development—with the greatest changes occurring in the critical first few weeks after your infant is born. The first milk your body produces, called colostrum, is a thick fluid with a yellow or orange tint that is low in volume but high in protein and easy for a newborn to digest. (If you deliver prematurely, your colostrum will contain even more protein and different types of fats that are important for premature babies.) After birth, colostrum gradually gives way to more mature milk, which is much greater in volume, lower in protein, and higher in lactose and fat, in accordance with your infant's evolving needs. The fat content of human milk changes during the course of a single feeding—starting out low in fat and increasing gradually throughout the feeding. The composition of mother's milk even changes over the course of the day.

Some studies have shown that scores on IQ and other cognitive ability tests of children who were breastfed as infants are higher than those of children who were fed formula, independent of socioeconomic factors or the mother's intelligence quotient. This increase is particularly striking among low-birthweight and premature infants. Of course, breastfeeding alone does not guarantee that your baby will be a child prodigy. But the evidence shows that in many aspects of infant development, being breastfed does offer the child a better chance of achieving her full genetic intellectual potential than formula-feeding does. Because a baby's brain develops at its most rapid rate during infancy and early childhood, the specific composition of human milk is important for developing the connections that enable brain cells to communicate with one another. Breastfeeding also enhances your baby's visual and auditory acuity, especially in premature infants.

∽ PSYCHOLOGICAL BENEFITS

Your newborn also benefits from the physical closeness of nursing. Thrust from the close, dark womb into an overwhelming experience of bright lights, loud noises, and new smells, your baby needs the reassurance of your continued physical presence. By holding him safe in your arms and giving nourishment from your body, you offer him a sense of continuity from pre- to post-birth life. Gazing into your eyes, your baby comes to understand that he is loved and protected and that you are there to provide for his needs as he adjusts to this new world. In addition, breastfeeding releases hormones in your body that promote mothering behaviors. This emotional bond is as vital as the nutritional benefit he receives from you. Scientists now tell us that infants learn best in a context of emotional closeness with an adult. Breastfeeding promotes a growing attachment between the two of you that will continue to play an important role in your baby's development for years to come.

IS BREASTFEEDING GOOD FOR ME TOO?

Breastfeeding is a wonderful gift for you as well. Many mothers feel fulfillment and joy from the physical and emotional communion they experience with their child while nursing. These feelings are augmented by the release of hormones such as prolactin, which produces a peaceful, nurturing sensation that allows you to relax and focus on your child, and oxytocin, which promotes a strong sense of love and attachment between the two of you. These pleasant feelings may be one of the reasons so many women who have breastfed their first child choose to breastfeed the children who follow.

Breastfeeding provides health benefits for mothers beyond emotional satisfaction. Mothers who breastfeed recover from

childbirth more quickly and easily. The hormone oxytocin, released during breastfeeding, acts to return the uterus to its regular
size more quickly and can reduce postpartum bleeding. Studies
show that women who have breastfed experience reduced rates of
breast and ovarian cancer later in life. Some studies have found
that breastfeeding may reduce the risk of developing type 2 diabetes, rheumatoid arthritis, and cardiovascular disease, including
high blood pressure and high cholesterol. Finally, exclusive breastfeeding delays the return of the mother's menstrual period, which
can help extend the time between pregnancies. (Exclusive breastfeeding can provide a natural form of contraception if the mother's

The Details on Calories

During lactation, women require an average of 400–500
additional calories per day to produce an adequate milk supply
for their baby. This exact amount will vary depending upon the
mother's pre-pregnancy weight, whether she is exclusively
breastfeeding, or whether she has begun to add solids to the
baby's diet. Some of the energy required to produce breast milk
comes from the mother's stores that were accumulated before
and/or during the pregnancy. Generally, the higher caloric
requirement occurs in the first six months of life. As the baby
gets older, beyond age six months, and begins eating solids, the
additional calories from the maternal diet begin to decrease.
Mothers who take in fewer calories while breastfeeding may
notice that they lose weight more quickly and those who
consume more calories will lose their pregnancy weight more
slowly. In general, slow, gradual weight loss after delivery and
during lactation is preferred to rapid weight loss.

menses have not returned, the baby is breastfeeding day and night, and the baby is less than six months old. See Chapter 6 for more information about breastfeeding and birth control.)

There are quite a few practical advantages to breastfeeding as well—bonuses the entire family can appreciate. For example, human milk is much less expensive than formula. During nursing you will need, at most, an extra 400 to 500 calories daily to produce sufficient milk for your baby, while formula can cost between $4 and $10 per day, depending upon the brand, type (powdered versus liquid), and amount consumed. At night, putting a baby to your breast is much simpler and faster than getting up to prepare or warm a bottle of formula. (Your partner can make night feedings even easier by changing the baby and bringing her to you for nursing.) It's wonderful, too, to be able to pick up the baby and go out—whether around town or on longer trips—without having to carry a bag full of feeding equipment. Breastfeeding is also good for the environment, since there are no bottles to wash or formula cans to throw away.

As welcome as all of these benefits are, though, most mothers put the feeling of maternal fulfillment at the top of their list of reasons for breastfeeding. Breastfeeding provides a unique emotional experience for the nursing mother and the baby. Breastfeeding is the one parenting behavior that only the mother can do for her baby, creating a unique and powerful physical and emotional connection. Your partner, the baby's siblings, and other relatives can all appreciate the new member of the family being welcomed in such a loving way.

IS FORMULA AN OPTION?

As scientists learn more about the composition of human milk, makers of formula continue to refine their product in an attempt to simulate its attributes as closely as possible. It is impossible to perfectly mimic a substance as complex as human milk, but formula does provide an alternative in cases where it's not possible to breastfeed exclusively or to provide expressed or donor human milk in a bottle.

A small percentage of new mothers are affected by physical conditions that interfere with milk production, such as insufficient development of the glands that produce milk (see Chapter 2) or the effects of breast reduction surgery. In the United States, women with the human immunodeficiency virus (HIV) are advised not to breastfeed, since the virus may be passed to their infant in the milk. Mothers newly diagnosed with infectious tuberculosis should not breastfeed directly unless they are on medication and no longer infectious. They can express their milk to be fed by another caregiver until they are no longer infectious. Breastfeeding is not advised while taking certain medications, such as illicit drugs and certain medications for severe psychiatric conditions. Any medication you take while nursing should be approved by your doctor. If the medication is not recommended while breastfeeding, your doctor may be able to offer you a safer alternative. Fortunately, most common medications can be taken by breastfeeding mothers. (See Chapter 5 for more information on medical conditions that may affect breastfeeding.)

The infant's medical condition, although less common, may preclude breastfeeding. Infants with a rare genetic disorder called galactosemia are unable to metabolize the sugar in human milk or standard cow's-milk-based formula. (Most states test for this condition as part of the newborn infant screen several days after birth.) Infants with the classic form of galactosemia must be fed a formula that does not contain lactose, or milk sugar. Extremely premature infants may be unable to breastfeed initially but can receive pumped milk. In some instances, the premature baby may require vitamin and mineral supplements, along with milk that the mother has expressed.

While medical issues that prohibit breastfeeding are uncommon, you may experience physical or psychological resistance to the process. Nursing your baby shouldn't hurt if your baby is attached (latched on) to the breast correctly, but incorrect attachment can cause nipple pain and even bleeding—particularly during the first few days of nursing. Some mothers feel discouraged by this negative early experience and are tempted to stop breastfeeding. However, in most cases, a hospital nurse, pediatrician, or lactation specialist can help you reposition your baby correctly at the breast and get nursing off to a much more comfortable start.

New mothers are also often strongly influenced by the advice and experiences of their partner, relatives, and friends. If your mother or other women close to you did not breastfeed their children or do not understand its benefits, they may encourage you to forgo breastfeeding and feed your baby formula instead. Your partner may also advocate formula-feeding. In most cases these loved ones mean well but are not well informed about the importance of breastfeeding. This book will provide you with answers to their questions or criticisms about breastfeeding and refer you to people in your community who will support whatever choice *you* make. If you find that you have become quite anxious about the breastfeeding experience—so much that your resistance may interfere with your relationship with your baby—it may help to talk to experienced breastfeeding mothers to allay your fears.

Certainly there is no reason to conclude that choosing any particular feeding plan makes you a good or bad parent. Still, barring any definite medical or physical problems that would interfere with lactation, it is advantageous to breastfeed. If you and your baby stay focused on the process and you have a good support system in place, most breastfeeding problems can be resolved within the first few weeks so you can settle into a comfortable breastfeeding relationship.

While at least twelve months is ideal, any amount of breastfeeding provides important benefits for you and your baby. If you worry that you will not be able to breastfeed after you return to work, it's still quite worthwhile to breastfeed until then. A few weeks before returning to work or school, you should experiment with using a breast pump, help your baby get used to taking expressed human milk from a bottle or alternative feeding method (see Chapter 9), and then reconsider whether it's really necessary to wean your child once you will be out of the house part of each day. Other solutions for continuing to breastfeed after return to work include nearby or on-site child care, flexible work hours, and job sharing.

BREASTFEEDING: A NATURAL GIFT

While the act of breastfeeding is entirely natural and has been done for centuries, you may be amazed by the resources that are in place these days to support it. At the urging of major health organizations, more health care providers are offering women the information and support they need to learn about breastfeeding. Local organizations have sprouted up to provide women with advice on the logistics of nursing. Some employers now provide lactation programs at on-site child care facilities, or at least offer access to appropriate facilities for using a breast pump to express milk. Most states have enacted laws to protect a mother's right to breastfeed in public places, and others cover benefits to protect a mother's right to continue to breastfeed or express her milk when she returns to work. Recognizing the importance of breastfeeding to the health of our nation, the United States has included many progressive strategies for breastfeeding in the workplace as part of health care reform. Examples of these provisions are that employers shall provide breastfeeding employees with "reasonable break time" and a private, non-bathroom place to express breast milk during the workday, up until the child's first birthday.

Even with all this support, most women have legitimate questions about breastfeeding. The following chapters are dedicated to helping you get ready for and experience your own breastfeeding journey, from preparing for those important early feedings to adjusting to home life, family life, and work life as a nursing mother and finally to moving with your child beyond breastfeeding. Hopefully, you will find that breastfeeding goes smoothly from the start. However, like anything new, it may take some time and practice to get the process going effectively. This is perfectly normal. In the meantime, stay positive and try not to get discouraged. Remember, your milk will provide your baby with more than just food. Breastfeeding is a wonderful natural gift that only you can give your baby, and we hope you will discover it to be a rewarding experience for both of you.

Q & A

How Will Breastfeeding Change My Life?

Q: *If I breastfeed, will I have to watch everything I eat, and do I have to drink milk all the time, as I did during pregnancy?*

A: In most cases you should maintain a healthy diet, as you would whether or not you were breastfeeding. (See Chapter 7 for more on nutrition.) One advantage of breastfeeding is that while you should eat an additional 400 to 500 calories per day, those calories add heft to your baby's thighs, not yours! You don't have to drink extra milk, since a breastfeeding mother's body efficiently absorbs calcium from other foods. In fact, you don't have to drink any cow's milk to make human milk. You do need a daily source of calcium in your diet, though, and will want to make sure your diet is adequate in vitamins and minerals. Consult your physician or your child's pediatrician if you're not sure that you are getting all the nutrients you need. A glass of wine or a cup of coffee is fine while nursing. In general, moderation is the key. In fact, a breastfeeding mother's diet is an excellent blueprint for a lifetime of healthy eating.

Q: *How can I manage to have free time to myself while breastfeeding on demand?*

A: During the first days after birth, all mothers, whether or not they breastfeed, must adjust to their babies' need for their almost constant presence. (This is usually not difficult, since you will want to get to know your baby and to rest and recuperate together.) Gradually, over the weeks that follow, you will find that you have an increasing amount of physical freedom. After the first few weeks, feedings will become more regular, giving you predictable times when you do not have to be present to breastfeed your child. With the proper preparation, your baby should be able to accept milk that you've expressed ahead of time and left for him in a bottle, if you choose to do so. If you wait until breastfeeding is well established, when your baby is at least three to four weeks old, this should not interfere with his ability to breastfeed. (See Chapter 9 for information on ways to prepare your baby to move from breast to bottle.) Remember to either breastfeed or express milk from your breasts the same number of times you would if you were with your baby all the time, about ten to twelve times per day. This will help to maintain your milk supply, a system that responds to the frequency and amount of milk removed from your breasts. This is also how many working mothers provide breast milk for their babies, enjoying the closeness of breastfeeding when at home while still affording the health benefits of human milk when they're away. In short, breastfeeding promotes physical closeness with your baby but does not mean you are tied to him constantly.

Q: *How can my partner be an active, involved parent if I'm breastfeeding exclusively?*

A: Just as your partner has already played a vital co-parenting role by supporting you during pregnancy and will continue to do so during childbirth, his parenting role will remain crucial as your baby makes the gradual transition from attachment to your body toward interaction with others in his world. There are many ways to be a parent besides feeding the baby. Your partner can provide you with nutritious meals so you can better feed your infant, help with household chores so you can rest, play with the baby during awake time, and rock him to sleep by holding him against his chest and singing in a low, soothing voice. If actually feeding the baby is important to your partner, he can offer your expressed milk in a bottle after the baby is at least several weeks old and has fully adjusted to the breast. (In Chapter 9 this process will be presented in greater detail, and in Chapter 11 we offer suggestions on many more ways in which your partner can fully participate in the parenting experience.) The bottom line, though, is that each parent's gifts to his child are different, but all are equally valuable.

CHAPTER 2

A Perfect Design:
How Breastfeeding Works

Breastfeeding is truly one of the marvels of nature. Like a beautifully choreographed dance, your body provides your baby with exactly what she needs, at the precise moment she needs it. The milk you produce sustains your baby with all the right nutrients, allowing her to grow and develop into a healthy child. Getting to the point where nursing is a natural part of your life is a slow, gradual process that begins with a complex interplay of hormones and changes in your breasts. It culminates with a successful nursing relationship between you and your infant. In this chapter, we'll take a close look at how this process unfolds and the changes you'll see in your body.

PREPARING TO BREASTFEED

Throughout your pregnancy, you will experience a number of physiologic changes preceding the birth of your baby. Many of these changes are preparing your body for the task of breastfeeding. Most notably, your breasts will increase in size as blood flow increases and the glandular tissue develops. But that increase doesn't happen overnight.

You probably noted early in your pregnancy—at around the fifth or sixth week—that your breasts had become fuller and your

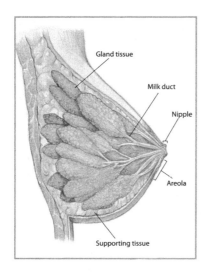

Gland tissue

Milk duct

Nipple

Areola

Supporting tissue

This schematic cross-section diagram of the breast shows that as your pregnancy progresses, the fatty and supportive tissues that normally make up most of the volume of the breast are replaced by glandular tissue necessary to produce milk.

nipples were more tender than before. Your nipples and the darker-colored area around them, called the *areolae,* may have enlarged and darkened, and the small bumps on the areolae, called *Montgomery's glands,* became more prominent. Starting about the third month of pregnancy, the complex interplay of a number of hormones—including prolactin, estrogen, progesterone, and human growth hormone—leads to the proliferation of milk ducts and gland-producing cells in your breasts as your body prepares for milk production.

As your pregnancy progresses, the glandular tissue necessary to produce milk replaces much of the fatty and supportive tissue that normally makes up most of the volume of your breast. This causes your breasts to become substantially larger during pregnancy and lactation. Such changes may worry you that breastfeeding will cause your breasts to sag or change shape after weaning, but there is no reason for concern. Once your baby is weaned from the breast (when you stop nursing and your milk glands are once again replaced by fatty and supportive tissue) and you return to your pre-pregnancy weight, your breasts will return to their approximate pre-pregnancy size and shape.

By the middle of your pregnancy, lactose—the sugar in milk—can be detected in your blood and urine, indicating that milk production is beginning. At the end of the second trimester, your body has become fully capable of producing milk—which means that even if your child is born prematurely, you will be able to produce it.

By the time you give birth, your milk-producing cells will have already begun the process of making the protein-rich colostrum that will start your baby on the road to good health. Colostrum is thick, somewhat sticky, and yellow or orange in color. (If you notice yellow or orange stains on the inside of your maternity bra, your breasts have already begun making colostrum. However, some mothers do not notice any colostrum being secreted until after their babies are born.) At this time, you may notice more prominent veins on the surface of your breasts and that the areolae have enlarged and become darker.

After your baby is born, the areolae of your breasts, and especially the nipples, will become exquisitely sensitive to touch. When your baby's mouth touches the nipple and areola, nerve cells will send a signal to your brain, causing the release of the hormone oxytocin. Oxytocin causes tiny muscle cells within the breasts to contract, squeezing milk from the milk-producing cells down the milk ducts toward the openings in the nipples. As your baby suckles at the breast, drawing milk through the nipple and into her mouth, the production of oxytocin will increase, causing more milk to be moved through the ducts in a process called the *let-down* or *milk ejection reflex.* The actual production of milk is maintained and regulated by prolactin, another hormone, especially in the early weeks of lactation. As breastfeeding progresses, sustained milk production becomes more dependent upon continued milk removal either by your baby nursing or by the expression of milk. This is a simplified description of the complex system by which your body ensures that whenever your infant is hungry, your body will provide her with the nourishment she needs.

Most women will notice a change in the volume of their breasts between the second and fifth days after giving birth. This change is the result of your milk "coming in." More frequent breastfeeding will help the milk come in more readily. In general, the process tends to occur later in women giving birth for the first time and earlier for those who have breastfed before. On subsequent days, you will feel your breasts getting fuller. After that, you may experience a week or two where your breasts will be very full with milk. If the fullness becomes extreme, it is called *engorgement*.

Many women who look forward to breastfeeding are concerned about whether their breasts are large enough to provide milk for their babies. While size may affect the volume of milk your breasts can hold at any given time—so that you may need to nurse more frequently if your breasts are smaller—breast size does not determine how much milk you make overall. As long as your baby is latched on and suckling correctly (see Chapter 4), the amount of milk you produce is determined by how much your baby nurses. The more milk she drinks, the more milk your body will produce. The less she breastfeeds, the less milk is produced.

AFTER CHILDBIRTH: WHAT HAPPENS NEXT?

As you will find, once you and your baby have settled into a comfortable nursing routine, breastfeeding relies on a wonderful pattern of supply and demand that ensures milk production in just the amounts your baby needs at any particular stage of growth. When your baby is especially hungry—in the second to third week of life, during growth spurts when he needs more calories, and so on—he will breastfeed more often, causing your milk production to increase so it can supply extra calories and nutrients. Increased nursing and even more fussiness at these times are normal and temporary. As he grows older and turns to other sources of food, your milk supply will gradually decrease. If at any time you want to increase or decrease the amount of milk you produce, all you need do is adjust the number and length of breastfeeding sessions.

COLOSTRUM: YOUR BABY'S FIRST MEAL

Colostrum provides all the nutrients and fluid that your newborn needs in the early days, as well as many substances to protect your baby against infections. Its color and thickness are due to the fact that it is higher in these protective factors. (Compared with more mature human milk, colostrum is also higher in protein, slightly lower in sugar, and significantly lower in fat.) While your breasts will not feel full the day that you give birth, you already have enough colostrum to nourish your baby. Your body will produce colostrum for several days after delivery until your milk increases in amount and becomes more creamy or white in color—a time that mothers frequently refer to as the milk "coming in."

Your baby will be born with a suckling instinct, though it is stronger in some babies than in others. Since this instinct is intense immediately after birth, it is best to introduce him to the breast within the first hour or so of life. Not only will his suckling at your breast stimulate your breasts to produce more milk, thus beginning the establishment of a reliable milk supply, but it will signal your uterus to contract and decrease the chance of excessive bleeding after delivery. This first feeding will also help him begin to learn how to nurse. Placing the newborn baby skin to skin against your chest will help to encourage your baby to smell the colostrum and want to latch on and begin his first feeding.

In fact, the initial phase of breastfeeding is a learning process for both mother and baby. Some newborns show little initial interest in nursing. Fortunately, newborns do not need much fluid, and their mothers' breasts contain only small amounts of the very important colostrum. At this stage, it is more important that babies feed frequently than it is for them to feed for long periods of time. Since the breasts are not yet extremely full of milk, they remain soft and supple after delivery, making it easier for the baby to learn to suckle.

In these early days, it is normal for a baby to lose some weight. This weight loss consists of extra fluid accumulated during pregnancy. In the days after delivery, your baby's appetite and need for fluids will increase. Approximately two to five days after birth, the colostrum production will give way to a higher volume of *transitional milk*.

TRANSITIONAL MILK

When breastfeeding mothers talk about their milk coming in, they are referring to the onset of production of transitional milk, the creamy milk that immediately follows colostrum. Transitional milk is produced anywhere from about two to five days after birth until ten to fourteen days after birth. Because your breasts will supply a much greater amount of transitional milk than colostrum, your breasts will become larger and firmer during this stage. This new fullness may feel uncomfortable at first and may make it more difficult for your baby to latch on to the breast correctly. With practice, however (and perhaps with the help of your baby's pediatrician or lactation specialist), you will help your baby latch on. Sometimes expressing a small amount of milk by hand will help to soften the areola enough to make it easier for the baby to latch. The drops of milk on your nipple also will encourage your baby to feed. Breastfeeding will ease the pressure in your breasts and make you feel more comfortable.

As your baby latches on and begins to breastfeed steadily, you may notice a tingly pins-and-needles sensation. This feeling tells you that the milk let-down reflex has occurred, causing milk to be pushed out of the milk-producing cells into milk ducts so it's available to your baby. The let-down reflex can be stimulated by your baby's suckling, an approaching feeding time, or just the sound of your baby's hungry cry. Once this happens, your milk will flow more plentifully and your baby will enjoy a satisfying feeding. You

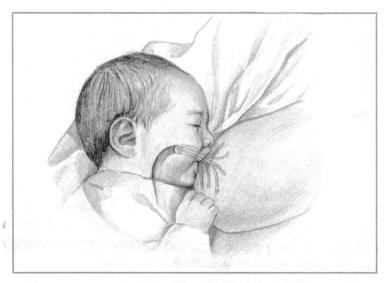

This baby is latched on properly with the tip of the nipple, shown schematically in cross section, deep within the baby's mouth.

will hear him swallowing more frequently. You may notice milk dripping or spurting from your other breast when let-down occurs. In the early weeks of breastfeeding, you may notice cramping or "afterpains" of your uterus when the baby feeds at the breast. This is yet another result of the hormone oxytocin. It is important for you to try to relax and rest, as stress, pain, and fatigue may decrease milk production and release.

The combination of sharply increased demand and the resulting increased human milk supply may make you feel like you are constantly breastfeeding during this early period. Daytime feedings may be anywhere from one and a half to three hours apart and may range in length from ten minutes to close to an hour each. Human milk is easily digested by the baby, and breastfed newborns typically nurse eight to twelve times a day. Soon, however, the nursing pattern will stabilize, and feedings will become less frequent. Over time, feedings will continue to change in frequency and length, depending upon your baby's needs.

MATURE MILK

In most women, mature milk begins to appear near the end of the second week after childbirth. Mature milk is produced in as great a volume as transitional milk but is thinner and more watery or even bluish; sometimes it's described as looking like skim milk when it is first secreted, until the fat is released later in the feeding and it becomes more creamy. Your breasts may appear somewhat softer and smaller than they did during the transitional-milk stage, though they will still be larger than before your pregnancy. These changes in your breasts and in your milk are normal and are designed to provide just what your baby needs for his nutrition, growth, and development.

Much later, after your baby begins to sample other liquids and solid foods, breastfeeding sessions will decrease in frequency. Some mothers choose to continue breastfeeding into the toddler or preschool years. By this time, the overall nutritional contribution of breastfeeding has diminished proportionate to the great variety of other beverages and solids the child is consuming. However, human milk continues to be as nutritious as cow's milk. The emotional and immunologic benefits of the nursing relationship continue throughout the period of lactation.

WHAT AFFECTS THE CONTENT OF MY BREAST MILK?

Pregnant women usually pay close attention to their diet, since every food, beverage, and drug they ingest may make its way to their baby. Fortunately, this is not exactly the case with breast milk. Milk is produced from the mammary glands in your breasts, not directly from the substances you ingest. These glands draw on the resources available in the form of nutrients from your diet and from your body's stores.

Still, breastfeeding requires extra energy and slightly different nutrient demands. A healthy nursing mother typically needs an additional 400 to 500 calories a day. This can be accomplished by a modest increase in a well-balanced diet. You should supplement your diet with calcium and vitamin D, either from foods or from a supplement. Taking a multivitamin/mineral supplement is a good insurance policy that both you and your baby are receiving good nutrition. Ideally, your diet should also include at least 200 milligrams of docosahexaenoic acid (DHA) to ensure that your baby gets DHA in the breast milk. DHA is a polyunsaturated omega-3 fatty acid that may improve your baby's visual and neurologic development. Eating just two portions of fish per week is enough to meet your and your baby's DHA needs. You should avoid eating certain types of fatty fish, such as pike, marlin, tilefish, shark, and swordfish, which tend to be higher in mercury. You may consider taking a DHA supplement if you eat a vegan diet that omits all animal products or if you don't eat fish.

If your diet contains insufficient calories or nutrients to fully sustain you and your nursing child, your mammary glands will have first shot at your body's available nutrients to produce highly nutritious human milk, leaving your body to rely on whatever is left over. So a less-than-ideal diet will probably not affect your breastfeeding child, but it may leave *your* body nutritionally depleted. (If you have any concerns that you may not be getting the proper amount of nutrients, talk to your doctor or a registered dietitian about improving your diet or the possibility of taking supplements.)

The mammary glands and cells that produce milk also help regulate how much of what you eat and drink actually reaches your baby. Some substances can affect your baby if you eat or drink too much of them. For instance, it's best to consume coffee, tea, and caffeinated sodas in moderation—probably no more than one or two cups of coffee a day—when you're breastfeeding. Caffeine tends to build up in babies' systems because they can't eliminate it easily. As a result, your baby may be irritable and sleep poorly. This may be more pronounced among premature babies. Some breastfeeding mothers are able to tolerate a larger intake of caffeine without any apparent effects upon their babies.

The American Academy of Pediatrics recommends that you limit the consumption of alcohol while you are breastfeeding. Alcohol can pass to your infant through your breast milk. If you do choose to have an occasional glass of wine or other alcoholic beverage, try to drink it just after you nurse rather than before. You should also drink alcohol with a meal to decrease the amount that is absorbed into your system. Waiting to breastfeed until several hours after consuming an alcoholic drink will help to ensure that the alcohol has passed through your system. If your breasts are uncomfortably full after drinking alcoholic beverages but it is too early to breastfeed your baby, you can pump and discard the milk. Keep in mind that some babies are more sensitive to what you eat and drink than others, so keep a close eye on your baby to see how she reacts to anything you ingest.

You also need to pay attention to the medications you take while you are nursing. It's reassuring to know that the drugs injected for epidural blocks and other types of regional anesthesia during childbirth do not pass into human milk sufficiently to cause long-term harm, though they may make your baby a little sleepy at first. If you are given general anesthesia (i.e., you are completely put to sleep), your anesthesiologist or obstetrician should be informed in advance of your plans to breastfeed. Generally, once you are awake and alert enough to breastfeed, then enough of the anesthetic drugs have cleared your system to make it safe for you to breastfeed.

While many medications are safe to take during breastfeeding, there are a few—including some nonprescription substances—that may be harmful to the baby. These are not always the same medications that are dangerous for pregnant women to ingest, so be sure to get approval for all medications from your doctor or your baby's pediatrician. You should not indulge in any kind of recreational drug, since enough of it could be passed on to your baby to cause serious harm. You also need to talk with your doctor if you are taking a drug that affects the mind, emotions, or behavior, known as psychotropic drugs. While many of these drugs are compatible with breastfeeding, there are others, including certain antidepressants, that may not be. For that reason, ask your health care professional to evaluate the medications you are taking and, if necessary, to recommend an alternative that is known to be safer while breastfeeding.

BREASTFEEDING METHODS: WHAT ARE MY ALTERNATIVES?

When most women imagine breastfeeding, they picture themselves nursing breast-to-mouth with their infant cradled in their arms. Certainly this is the most common form of breastfeeding, and because it affords physical contact and an emotional connection for mother and baby, it is the most fully satisfying form. However, if you are unable to directly nurse your baby for medical reasons (your baby is born premature or you have a serious illness yourself) or practical ones (your temporary absence), alternative methods of giving your child human milk are available. In Chapter 9, you will learn how to use a manual or electric breast pump to express milk from your breasts and store it in the refrigerator or freezer for later use. Expressed milk can be fed to any baby whose mother is away at work, at school, shopping, or absent for other reasons. It can be fed to a premature baby with a dropper, spoon, or bottle and to an older baby in a bottle or cup. As your baby gets older, your partner can feed him with your expressed milk to share in the feeding process or let you get some extra sleep. Throughout this book, you will find plenty of ways to provide your baby with human milk in one form or another.

The small percentage of mothers who cannot use their own milk to feed their babies may have the option of obtaining other mothers' processed, pasteurized human milk that has been donated to milk banks in much the same way that blood is commonly donated. Donated human milk does not provide full protection against diseases in the environment, since it must be heat-treated to destroy any potentially dangerous bacteria, viruses, or other infectious particles, but it does provide some of the immune benefits and many of the nutrients that formula does not supply.

EMPOWERING YOURSELF

Breastfeeding is not a static process. From the moment you become pregnant to the time you are nursing your infant, your body undergoes a series of changes, all designed to support your decision to breastfeed. Understanding your breasts and how they nourish your child can help you gain the confidence you need as you embark on your own breastfeeding journey. While there is nothing like experience to help you truly understand the process of breastfeeding, you can learn as much as you can ahead of time by reading books like this one, talking to other breastfeeding moms and lactation specialists, and exploring the Internet. Soon breastfeeding will become a rewarding part of your life and the life of your growing baby.

CHAPTER 3

Getting Ready for Your Baby

By now, you may have already made the decision: you're going to breastfeed your baby. In fact, approximately 75 percent of women make their infant feeding decision either before they became pregnant or during the first trimester. Even with that amount of certainty, however, you may still have questions regarding the details of breastfeeding. How will you know when your baby has had enough to eat? Is it okay to let your baby drift off to sleep while nursing? Are you worried that you will not be able to produce enough milk for your baby?

If you're feeling overwhelmed with questions and concerns—and not just about nursing—join the club. Most pregnant women have lots of questions! The key to getting them answered is locating the right resources before delivering your baby. That means visiting your obstetrician for a breast exam, attending breastfeeding classes, and putting together a network of post-childbirth support that includes friends and family members. All of this preparation will help ensure breastfeeding success before your baby is born. It also helps to pay attention to practical matters—such as health insurance coverage, child care issues, and your plan for breastfeeding at the workplace—ahead of time, so you can focus on your baby after the birth. In this chapter, you will find a number of ways to get ready for your baby, to educate yourself as fully as possible about how breastfeeding works, and to put together an optimal support team to help you with any questions that come up later.

The better you lay the groundwork now, the more you and your baby will benefit.

CAN I BREASTFEED? PREPARING YOUR BODY FOR NURSING

Breastfeeding is a natural process that requires no special physical preparation for most women. However, you should discuss your plans to breastfeed with your obstetrician/gynecologist and have him examine your breasts as early as possible in your pregnancy and again during the third trimester. Tell him about any breast-feeding or early weaning problems you've had with previous children, or of any breast biopsies, implants, reductions, or other breast surgeries you've experienced. Let him know if you have or have had any rashes on the breast or nipples, lumps involving your breasts, or infections. Also, make sure he knows of any chronic medical problems or illnesses you have, such as HIV infection, breast lesions, depression, or diabetes. Chances are excellent that he will tell you he foresees no trouble in your ability to produce enough milk for your baby, even if you have experienced one or more of these situations. (See Chapter 5 for more information about the effects of breast surgery on nursing.) However, if you have had problems before or the condition of your breasts suggests special challenges ahead, being aware of these potential challenges can make all the difference in your ability to successfully breast-feed.

As discussed in Chapter 2, small breast size does not predict an insufficient milk supply for the baby. In fact, the size of a woman's breast before pregnancy is determined by the supporting structures and not the actual glandular tissue. So the size of the breast does not affect the ability of the breast to produce adequate milk to nourish an infant. While breast size does not affect the volume of milk that can be produced, it does have some impact on storage capacity for milk. As a result, women with smaller breasts may find they need to breastfeed their infants more often, while women with larger breasts may find their babies will go somewhat longer between feedings.

All women should experience increased breast size during pregnancy. These breast changes are good signs that the glandular tissue is present and responding to the maternal hormones of pregnancy. Women whose breasts do not enlarge at least somewhat during pregnancy (regardless of their pre-pregnancy breast size) may experience difficulty in producing sufficient milk. This is not the case for every mother whose breasts remain relatively unchanged, but it is a caution sign your obstetrician should note on your prenatal record and communicate to your pediatrician, lactation specialist, and other medical personnel. This helps ensure that your baby's milk intake will be monitored carefully to see that she is getting enough nourishment.

Your obstetrician should note other variations in breast size or shape. Large breasts can make it awkward to hold the baby in a correct position to nurse, or make it hard for the baby to latch on to the breast. Breasts of markedly unequal size may lead to a normal supply of milk in one breast but little milk produced by the other; however, women can produce adequate milk for their baby by feeding from only one breast. Extremely small or abnormally shaped breasts sometimes contain an insufficient number of milk glands; breastfeeding in these cases should be closely monitored to be sure enough milk is being produced. It is important to understand that none of these characteristics means that you will be unable to breastfeed successfully. They simply mean that your health care professionals should pay particularly close attention to early breastfeeding, make sure everything is proceeding smoothly, and offer you solutions to any problems that arise.

⌒ INVERTED OR FLAT NIPPLES

One breast characteristic you should certainly point out to your obstetrician and pediatrician is inverted or flat nipples. Inverted

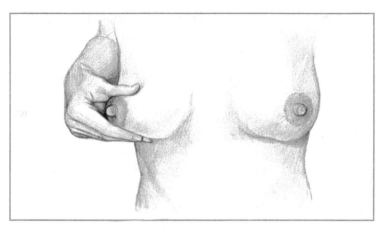

A normally protruding—or everted—nipple becomes erect when you press the areola between two fingers.

nipples retract inward toward the breast instead of protruding out when the areola is gently squeezed. Flat nipples neither retract nor protrude but remain more or less flat. When not compressed, some inverted nipples appear normal. Others contain a small dimple or may have a clear indentation at all times. You can test your own nipples by gently compressing the areola about one to two inches

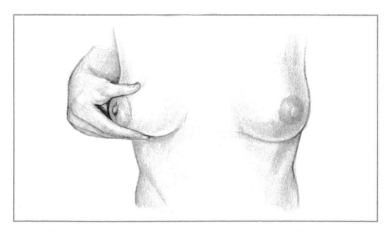

Inverted nipples retract toward the breast when pressure is applied to the areola.

behind the nipple. If your nipples draw inward or remain flat, tell your obstetrician and pediatrician.

Inverted nipples, and to a lesser extent flat nipples, can create a problem during breastfeeding by making it more difficult for the baby to properly latch on to the breast. In some cases, inverted nipples may actually impede the flow of milk. They are also more prone to injury of the nipple surface. Fortunately, a woman with inverted or flat nipples can still breastfeed if her nipples can protrude outward with stimulation. In addition, inverted and flat nipples sometimes become sufficiently everted, or normally protruding, on their own during pregnancy, so that by the time the baby is born, breastfeeding can proceed without problems. Even if the nipples don't evert on their own, this characteristic should not prevent most women from successfully breastfeeding their children. Solutions to this relatively common problem are in Chapter 4.

Some methods used in the past to correct inverted nipples during pregnancy may actually reduce breastfeeding success and are no longer routinely recommended. These include using breast shells—plastic cups with a hole in the center that are pressed against the breasts, leaving the nipples exposed. (Breast shells may

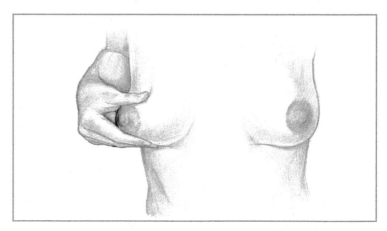

Flat nipples neither retract nor protrude, remaining more or less flat.

Pierced Nipples

In most cases, pierced nipples do not interfere with breastfeeding, though any rings or studs should be removed prior to a breastfeeding session to prevent choking. If your piercing became infected at the time of the piercing or later, inform your doctor. Such infection, as well as any scarring that may have occurred, can make nursing more difficult. While breastfeeding, some of your milk may leak through the pierced hole. This is usually not a problem, but if you have any questions, be sure to ask your pediatrician or a lactation specialist to check that your baby is nursing well.

be helpful after childbirth, although their benefit has not been proven in studies. See Chapter 4.) Manual exercises to encourage the nipples to protrude, called nipple rolling, have no effect. Experts now agree that it is best to wait until after childbirth to address inverted nipples—but your medical support team certainly should be informed about your situation to better guide you.

CHANGES IN YOUR BREASTS

As was noted in the previous chapter, physical changes in your breasts will occur as your pregnancy continues and your body prepares for nursing. Your breasts will grow larger and may begin to secrete colostrum. These scant secretions can leave yellow stains on your clothing. In rare cases, the stains may be rust-colored or brown. This means they may contain dried blood —also usually a result of normal breast development—but do mention this to your obstetrician.

Many women experience a new tenderness in their nipples.

This is a normal aspect of pregnancy as well, though sometimes it can be exacerbated by a dry climate or rough-textured clothing worn next to the skin. In the past, experts may have encouraged expectant mothers to use creams, lotions, "toughening-up" exercises, and other techniques to decrease nipple sensitivity and prepare for nursing, but it is now understood that nature offers the best preparation. In fact, your body secretes a lubricating substance through small, raised areas on the areola called Montgomery's glands. Usually this is all that's needed to prevent undue dryness. If you find that your nipples continue to feel extremely sensitive, dry, and flaky as childbirth approaches, try keeping them uncovered for an hour or more a day. If that doesn't work, apply a small amount of medical-grade lanolin, labeled as purified (available at most pharmacies or through a lactation specialist).

⟨⟩ MEDICATION

At the time of your breast exam or as soon as possible after you have learned that you are pregnant, inform your obstetrician about any medications you are currently taking or know you will be taking after childbirth. She will be able to tell you if your medication is safe during breastfeeding and may be able to provide you with a safe substitute if it is not. You may also be prescribed a shorter-acting form of the medication, advised to take the drug right after breastfeeding, and told to monitor your baby for any adverse effects.

If you are told that you cannot breastfeed while taking a particular drug, consider getting a second opinion. (Many professionals are unsure about issues of drugs in breast milk and prefer to err on the side of caution.) It is important to clear up any confusion long before your due date approaches. The hospital staff may be uncomfortable with you breastfeeding if they are unfamiliar with whether the medications you are taking can be safely used during lactation.

Can I Breastfeed Too?

PREPARING FOR YOUR ADOPTED BABY

If you are adopting a newborn or older baby in the near future, you may know of adoptive mothers who breastfed their children and wonder whether you might do the same.

You will find more detailed information about adoptive breastfeeding in Chapter 5. In the meantime, if you are considering this, talk with your doctor and pediatrician, as well as a lactation specialist, or your local La Leche League representative. They can help you assess your specific situation and your future baby's needs, instruct you on how to stimulate milk production, teach you how to supplement feedings with donated human milk or formula, and even put you in touch with other adoptive mothers who have successfully breastfed. Since induced lactation works best with a newborn or a very young baby, it's best to research this issue sooner rather than later. Ideally, you will want to begin inducing lactation weeks to months before your baby arrives.

WHAT ELSE DO I NEED TO KNOW? GATHERING INFORMATION ABOUT BREASTFEEDING

You and your partner will benefit greatly by taking time before your baby's birth to learn all you can about the mechanics of breastfeeding. Books, such as this one, can answer many of your questions; videos may also be helpful. The fact is, though, that with breastfeeding, nothing beats personal guidance from an expert. We recommend, if possible, taking a breastfeeding course that lasts for several sessions.

Your obstetrician or pediatrician may be able to refer you to a good breastfeeding course in your area. Hospitals frequently provide such courses and may offer private consultations with a lactation specialist as well. Another option is to attend meetings offered by La Leche League International, a nonprofit organization with chapters in nearly every American city. La Leche League, founded in the 1950s by a group of Chicago mothers who saw a need for mother-to-mother support in breastfeeding, provides nursing women with individual help through breastfeeding meetings, in-person and telephone counseling, informative publications, information via the Internet, and even special equipment when necessary. Many couples appreciate that all La Leche League counselors—including those who conduct instructional meetings—are experienced mothers who have themselves breastfed. They understand exactly what new mothers are going through. Attending the meetings before you give birth will help you familiarize yourself with what other services your local group offers and decide whether this approach suits your personal philosophy and style. (See contact information in Appendix 1.)

Government initiatives such as the WIC program (the Special Supplemental Nutrition Program for Women, Infants, and Children) also offer breastfeeding courses or counseling. The WIC program, operated by the U.S. Department of Agriculture in partnership with state and local health departments, provides other services as well—including one-on-one prenatal breastfeeding education, nutrition information, health care referrals, postpartum follow-up and counseling, peer support programs, and extra food—to families whose income is below a certain level. The maximum allowable income changes from year to year but is not as low as might be expected. About 63 percent of all infants born in the United States in 2006 were eligible for WIC, and, of those eligible, about three-fourths were participating in the program. To find out whether you qualify, call your local or state health department, listed in your local phone book, or see Appendix 1.

What a Course Can't Cover

Breastfeeding courses cover a wide array of situations that new parents experience, but if your particular circumstances require additional help, you may need to dig further for information. Parents expecting twins or greater multiples, for example, should contact a local chapter of the National Organization of Mothers of Twins Clubs (see Appendix 1) for advice on how to breastfeed multiples, what (if any) special equipment you may need, and what kind of extra help you may want to secure for your return home after birth. Since there is a greater chance that your babies may be born prematurely, you should also find out how to provide your infants with milk if they are unable to nurse at first. (See Chapter 5.) If you know your baby will be born with a birth defect, such as a cleft palate, heart defect, or other medical problem that may affect her ability to nurse, dedicate some time now to researching your child's condition and contacting appropriate support groups (see Appendix 1).

If you suffer from a medical problem such as chronic depression, anxiety disorder, hepatitis, tuberculosis, or any infectious disease that may prevent you from nursing, discuss the issue as soon as possible with your pediatrician, obstetrician, and the doctor who is treating you for the illness. Most medical conditions are compatible with breastfeeding, but you will want to be sure.

All parents who expect to confront a special situation regarding breastfeeding should discuss the issue with their obstetrician and their child's pediatrician before the birth. Your doctor can refer you to a lactation specialist (or one may be available at the hospital where you will give birth) who can talk with you about how to successfully breastfeed. Your La Leche

League contact can also provide you with valuable advice, support, and references in all of these areas and can in most cases put you in touch with other mothers who have breastfed successfully under similar circumstances.

Attending breastfeeding classes makes at least as much sense as partaking in a more traditional childbirth course, since you will spend more time breastfeeding than you will giving birth. Breastfeeding instruction is even more important now that your hospital stay after delivery can be as short as twenty-four to forty-eight hours. By attending a class and preparing in other ways, you can ensure that you will be reasonably well informed long before you arrive at the hospital. Be sure to ask anyone else who expects to help you begin breastfeeding to attend these classes as well, to learn how best to support you and your baby, and to explore their role as a non-breastfeeding caregiver.

WHO WILL BE THERE IF I NEED HELP? CREATING A NETWORK OF POSTPARTUM SUPPORT

In traditional societies, new mothers have always relied on other, experienced women to help them with the most common questions and concerns regarding breastfeeding. Growing up watching mothers nurse their babies makes it easier to learn to breastfeed, but even if a woman has never seen breastfeeding, she can benefit by finding other experienced nursing mothers to support her. Today in this country, we also have the knowledgeable assistance of such trained experts as pediatricians, hospital nurses, lactation specialists, and La Leche League volunteers. Since breastfeeding is a learned skill, not an instinctive process, such advice is always helpful. If you have trouble establishing a nursing pattern after childbirth, you may find it indispensable.

☞ THE RIGHT HOSPITAL

To ensure a successful start for breastfeeding, it is helpful to give birth in a breastfeeding-friendly location—a place where mothers are encouraged to stay with their newborns around the clock (called *rooming-in*) and babies are not offered pacifiers or supplemental feedings that will interfere with their ability to nurse. In recent years many hospitals have become more active in this regard as the demand for breastfeeding has increased, but be sure to check on your hospital or birthing center before delivery.

Tour the hospitals that are available to you and ask your tour guide what the facility's maternity policies are. Does this hospital officially encourage breastfeeding on demand, and are all health staff instructed to implement and support this policy? Are mothers and babies kept together immediately after birth and helped to initiate breastfeeding shortly after birth? Are supplemental feedings given only for medical reasons or if the mother has requested it? Are babies allowed to stay in the mother's room full-time? Ask whether the hospital or birthing center maintains one or more lactation specialists on staff and whether the regular nursing staff both supports breastfeeding and spends time helping new mothers learn to nurse. Are breastfeeding classes available both before and after delivery? Finally, find out whether they routinely refer new mothers to breastfeeding support groups in the area and other sources of postpartum help.

Some hospitals and birthing centers in the United States have been certified as Baby-Friendly Hospitals, which means that the hospital has complied with a specified ten-step process of training, education, and support to provide breastfeeding mothers and babies with the best start in breastfeeding. The Baby-Friendly Hospital

Initiative, developed internationally by UNICEF, the World Health Organization, and other organizations such as Wellstart International, is administered in the United States by Baby-Friendly USA.

Your choice of a hospital or birthing center may be limited by geographic location, insurance or HMO coverage, and doctor-hospital affiliations. Inspecting busy hospitals can sometimes be intimidating. Keep in mind, however, that childbirth is a competitive market in this country and your business is wanted. Choose a facility with which you feel comfortable and whose staff will help you begin your life with your baby in the way you know is best. Find out where your obstetrician has privileges, since that will determine where he delivers patients.

∞   THE RIGHT PEDIATRICIAN

Another invaluable source of breastfeeding support in the period immediately following childbirth is your child's pediatrician. Since this medical professional may need to make decisions regarding feedings immediately after childbirth, when you may or may not be able to participate depending on your medical condition, it is important to choose the most appropriate person ahead of time and communicate your plans for breastfeeding.

The best way to create a "short list" of potential pediatricians is to solicit recommendations from friends with babies or young children, from your obstetrician, from your hospital or birthing center, through online resources, and from the volunteers at your local La Leche League. Once you've solicited several names, consider scheduling a prenatal visit with each candidate, selecting one who inspires your confidence and with whom you feel a personal comfort. Be sure he is knowledgeable and supportive of breastfeeding practices, aware of any potential problems you have discovered, and willing to support your efforts to nurse from the beginning. You might want to ask the pediatrician the following questions—but be sure to customize this list to suit your own needs.

- What percentage of the infants in your practice are breastfed?
- How soon after birth do you recommend that a mother begin breastfeeding?
- What is your opinion regarding rooming-in for mother and baby?
- How long do you typically recommend exclusive breastfeeding?
- About how long do most of the mothers in your practice breastfeed?
- How will I be able to tell if my breastfed baby is getting enough milk and growing properly?
- Is there an age at which you recommend weaning?
- What advice do you provide to breastfeeding mothers about returning to work?

You can also ask your pediatrician about breastfeeding classes in the community, books and videos that might be worth purchasing or borrowing, and names of lactation specialists. Don't hesitate to ask for time just to talk. Pediatricians understand that it's important for parents to find an appropriate caregiver for their child. Few patient-doctor matches are absolutely perfect, but you should feel a certain amount of personal ease with your child's doctor. If you choose a family physician to care for your child, the same selection process would apply.

∞   MORE BREASTFEEDING SUPPORT

You can secure support from professionals trained specifically in breastfeeding practices even before you have your baby. These advisers—baby nurses, doulas (women who care for the mother during labor, delivery, and after childbirth so the mother can focus on her baby), and lactation specialists—may be recommended by your obstetrician, made available by your hospital or birthing center, or even suggested by other mothers who have benefited from their services.

Lactation specialists come from a variety of backgrounds. Many are nurses with special expertise in mother-baby care. Others are certified IBCLCs (International Board Certified Lactation Consultants) who have completed course work, logged a specific amount of clinical practice hours, and passed a standardized exam that covers infant feeding, breast anatomy, milk production, management of breastfeeding complications, and stages of infant development. Unlike a nurse or physician, the IBCLC designation alone does not mean a person is licensed by the state to practice as a health care professional, but most IBCLCs do have a great deal of experience working with breastfeeding mothers. It's a good idea to interview a potential lactation specialist before the birth, if possible, to discuss such issues as training, number of nursing mothers assisted, fee structures, references, and the possibility and frequency of post-partum visits to your home or at her office. You might also inquire about backup arrangements in case she is unavailable.

ᗡ   FAMILY SUPPORT

Ideally, by your due date you will have formed relationships with one or more of the following: a pediatrician or other pediatric health care provider, members of your local La Leche League and/or WIC office, and perhaps a doula, baby nurse, or lactation specialist. Now is also the time to assemble the family members and friends whom you expect to support you in this new venture. Talk with your baby's father about how he can make it possible for you to focus on the baby during the vital first weeks of breastfeeding. (See Chapter 11 for ideas about this.) Talk with your older children, if you have any, in a matter-of-fact way about how you will breastfeed this baby and what they might do to help. (More information about older siblings is also available in Chapter 6.) Welcome offers from other family members to help as long as they understand and support your determination to breastfeed. Well-meaning friends and loved ones believe they are helping when they offer to give the baby a bottle or ignore the baby's demands for a feeding to "let you get some rest." But you will not want or need anyone, no matter how close, to discourage you from getting breastfeeding off to a good start. If you feel this may happen, provide your helper with other activities (washing dishes, doing laundry, changing the baby's diaper, or playing with her) that can help you get some rest, or ask her to visit a couple of months after the birth, when your nursing routine has been established.

IS THE PAPERWORK DONE?

While you are pregnant, it's important to take care of any practical chores relating to breastfeeding. Before you leave work on maternity leave, for example, you will want to talk with your employer and determine how you can provide human milk for your baby after your return. In Chapter 10 you will find information on how to secure a private space and regular breaks for expressing human milk on the job, and you'll learn how to store your milk so your child's caregiver can feed it to him in a bottle or cup. By reviewing this information before the birth, you can make a plan that best suits your work and home situations. It's best to put your agreement in writing with your employer before you leave to have your baby, so you'll feel more confident about your return to work and your employer will be reassured that you do intend to return.

While you are thinking about your return to work, you may also give some thought to how well your baby's caregiver or child care center will follow the practices and instructions you set for feeding your baby. (This issue is discussed at greater length in Chapter 9.) If you are currently in the process of choosing a caregiver or child care program, you will need to discuss your breastfeeding plans in the interview or conversation. Your baby's caregivers must be comfortable with the idea of handling bottles filled with your milk, for example, and must agree to follow your directions regarding formula supplements, whether and when to introduce solid foods, and so on. Bring up the relevant issues during your first talks with a potential caregiver, rather than waiting until the weeks or days before you return to your job.

Since you may require the services of a lactation specialist or need to rent a breast pump or other breastfeeding equipment after your baby is born, review your health care policy now to see if it covers such services. If these costs will not be reimbursed, consider budgeting for what you might need or talk to your plan administrator about getting breastfeeding services covered. Many insurance companies are now aware of the many health benefits and the decreased health care costs associated with breastfeeding and are interested in investing in services that support breastfeeding. Be sure you have identified any community resources that will provide you with breastfeeding help should the need arise. There are a growing number of companies that provide lactation support services in the workplace, because it has been demonstrated that women who breastfeed when they return to work actually save the company money through fewer missed days of work, fewer doctor visits for illness, fewer hospitalizations, and reduced use of prescription medications. Find out what breastfeeding support your workplace might provide.

One final bit of paperwork involves your plan for exclusively breastfeeding your baby while still at the hospital. While most hospital policies have made progress toward supporting exclusive breastfeeding, ask your obstetrician to include specific instruction in your birthing plan regarding your desire to avoid feeding supplements for your baby and to keep him with you in your room. Studies have shown that newborns adjust most easily to breastfeeding when they are not provided with alternatives such as formula, water, or even pacifiers. Also inform your partner or other birthing coach about your desire to breastfeed soon after childbirth, and remind your obstetrician and obstetrical nurses about this, if possible, early in your labor.

WHAT DO I NEED TO BREASTFEED?
OPTIONAL AIDS TO MAKE NURSING EASIER

Throughout most of human history, mothers have successfully breastfed their babies without the help of nursing pillows, breast pads, or even rocking chairs. Our bodies, and our children's bodies, are well designed to make nursing a simple and rewarding process. Still, some supplies can make life as a nursing mother easier, if they fit into your budget. (Nursing equipment also makes wonderful baby gifts.)

A well-made nursing bra that comfortably supports your enlarged breasts can be useful. It is difficult to predict what size nursing bra you will need, but take your best guess and purchase at least one or two while pregnant to have for the hospital. After childbirth you can be fitted for one, which should never be tight or constricting. Nursing bras have front flaps that can be detached with one hand (while the other is supporting the baby) and pulled open for nursing. Outer clothing designed for nursing provides openings for the baby to access the breast and is a practical idea for mothers

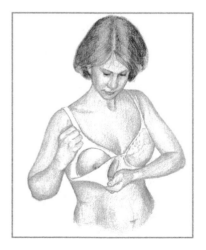

Nursing bras provide proper support and have front flaps that can be detached with one hand.

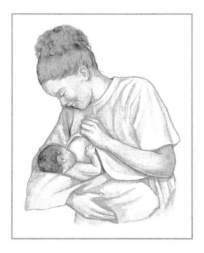

Shirts that can be lifted with one hand make nursing easier.

concerned about nursing discreetly in public. Both nursing bras and clothing are available at maternity shops, in mother-child clothing catalogs, and at many department stores. Of course, shirts that can easily be lifted up and blouses that unbutton from the bottom up also work quite well.

Disposable or washable breast pads, which can be slipped inside the bra cup to absorb any milk that leaks out between feedings, are useful for women whose breasts leak a great deal or who sometimes find themselves away from their babies at a regular feeding time. Avoid pads with plastic liners that impede the flow of air around the nipples and hold the moisture in, which can irritate the nipples. Breast pads can be purchased at most pharmacies and grocery stores—though a folded piece of absorbent cloth works almost as well.

While not necessary for successful breastfeeding, equipment to help you hold, cuddle, and soothe your baby can be a welcome addition to a nursery. Some mothers find that a custom-made nursing pillow, designed to help you position your baby properly and hold her for an entire feeding without tiring your arms, is easier than trying to arrange ordinary pillows or cushions. (Nursing pil-

Packing Your Bag

WHAT TO TAKE TO THE HOSPITAL

While the average hospital stay for a new mother and baby has decreased significantly over recent years, there's still no way to predict whether you will be away from home for a day or for a week. So it's a good idea to pack some breastfeeding supplies along with your toiletry bag and a list of friends and relatives to call.

The nursing bras you bought during your pregnancy are definite items to put into the suitcase. While you might not wear them during your hospital stay, you can check the fit after childbirth, or practice unhooking the front flap one-handed before you nurse. A nightgown with slits at the breasts for easy, discreet nursing is also helpful when you expect visitors outside your immediate family, though with practice you will soon find it easy to breastfeed with reasonable modesty even with non-nursing clothes. Some women pack breast pads, though these are rarely necessary in the early days, when the amount of colostrum or milk being produced is small and leaking is uncommon. Nursing pillows to support the baby while breastfeeding and medical-grade lanolin to soothe tender nipples may not be necessary this early in the process—but if it reassures you to know they'll be nearby, by all means bring them. And pack this book as well; at two in the morning, when your partner is asleep and the lactation specialist is not available, you may find answers to your most urgent questions here.

lows come in various shapes and sizes, so you may want to try out several before choosing one that suits you.) A footstool raises the level of your lap, bringing your baby closer to your breast. It also helps keep your back straight, which may make you more comfortable. Some new mothers enjoy a rocking chair or glider to use in the baby's room in anticipation of those precious moments when a nursing session blends into sleep.

Other pieces of optional equipment include a baby sling or carrier that frees your hands while keeping your baby close enough to nurse, and a bassinet for keeping your sleeping infant beside your bed. You can find these items in most baby supply stores and baby equipment catalogs. Please remember, however, that special equipment and furnishings are all extras. All you really need to nurse successfully are your breasts and a hungry baby.

THE BIG DAY

Making preparations to breastfeed, and learning as much as you can beforehand, can help you transition more easily into your role as a nursing mother. It's also important to line up people who will support your decision to nurse and have experts around to answer your questions and concerns, whether it is your baby's pediatrician, your obstetrican, or a lactation specialist. Make sure you keep your partner involved in this decision-making process, as this support is of paramount importance to your success as a breastfeeding mother.

Now is the time for you to prepare the best possible environment for your baby's arrival, with a hospital that encourages you to breastfeed and loving support from family and friends. Breastfeeding is a natural process, but it always begins more easily with a little help from professionals, relatives, and friends. For many new mothers, the first few weeks after childbirth pass in an exciting blur. The more preparation you do before the baby's birth, the easier it will be to care for and breastfeed your baby after the birth.

CHAPTER 4

The First Feedings

As any mom can tell you—and perhaps you already know—planning the delivery of your baby is virtually impossible. Most babies don't arrive on their due dates, and every delivery story is unique. Some women labor for hours, while others give birth relatively quickly. But in the midst of all the activity, you'll want to remain focused on breastfeeding your baby as soon as you can after delivery. Those early feedings will help set the stage for your next few months—maybe even years—of breastfeeding.

FIRST ENCOUNTER

The minutes following childbirth are typically an exciting time for everyone involved. As you recover from your physical experience of labor and delivery, you may feel overwhelmed by an enormous number of new feelings, hopes, and uncertainties. Of course, this is also a time when you want the professional treatment of your newborn to proceed according to your wishes. Ideally, you will have informed your obstetrician and pediatrician ahead of time of your desire to breastfeed, as recommended in Chapter 3. Your partner or birthing coach should remind your pediatrician and obstetrical or newborn nurses that you do not want your baby to be given water, a pacifier, or supplemental feedings without a valid medical reason.

Ideally, you will want your baby placed on your abdomen moments after delivery. You will want to breastfeed within an hour or so of giving birth to take advantage of your baby's suckling instinct. When placed in skin-to-skin contact with the mother, the alert, healthy infant is capable of latching on to the breast without specific assistance within the first hour after birth. Infants who are placed on their mother's abdomen after birth and who attach to the breast within an hour have more successful breastfeeding experiences than infants who do not attach early on. Milk let-down also occurs earlier in mothers who breastfeed their infants soon after birth. In fact, babies who nurse early after delivery are more likely to still be breastfeeding at two to four months of age than infants who start nursing more than two hours after birth. Immediate breastfeeding also starts the process of establishing your future milk supply and helps your uterus contract and return to its pre-pregnancy state, which decreases the chance of excessive bleeding after delivery.

Breastfeeding immediately is possible with most healthy births,

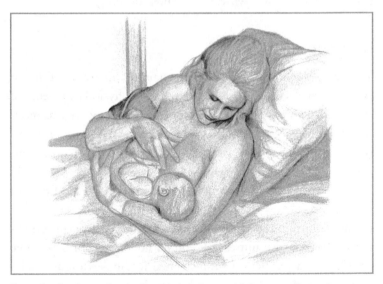

Breastfeeding immediately after birth helps establish your milk supply and encourages your baby's natural instinct to nurse.

when a baby needs little medical care beyond drying off and keeping warm. Offering your breast to your infant at this time will help her take advantage of her natural instincts to latch on and suckle. You should place your baby in skin-to-skin contact on your abdomen or chest, with bare skin against bare skin. Have your baby wear nothing, except a diaper if you prefer. If the baby is cold, your temperature will increase to bring the baby's temperature up. This skin-to-skin placement will also allow the baby direct access to the breast.

This is not to say that your newborn will instantly know what to do. Some mothers find that their babies do not actively suckle during the first few attempts but instead simply snuggle contentedly against the breast, tentatively lick the nipple, or attach to the breast and suckle briefly but then stop and look around. Many others find that their babies latch on right away and suckle as if they've been doing it for months. (Most babies have already been practicing by sucking on their fingers or arms in the uterus.) Whether or not your infant actually breastfeeds productively at this time is not critical. Rather, this is a time for the two of you to start to get to know each other, for her to be introduced to the breast, and for her to begin to associate the sight, smell, and feel of your breasts with the satiety of her hunger and thirst. She also learns that being held skin to skin makes her feel warm, comfortable, and nurtured.

This first feeding is important for you, too, in that it represents your first step in establishing a breastfeeding relationship. No matter how well you have prepared ahead of time, your first real breastfeeding experience may feel a little strange. Your baby's tongue on your nipple or her firm grip on your breast may feel different from what you'd imagined, or you may find that you are unsure whether you are holding her correctly or whether she's truly latched on. You may perceive help from nurses as intrusive or feel self-conscious trying to breastfeed in a room full of strangers. All of these feelings are normal for a new mother. As in any partnership, you and your newborn will have to learn and adjust to each other's style. As with any physical skill, mastery will come with practice. For now it's best to relax, enjoy this moment, and wait until you've both had some rest before worrying about perfecting your technique.

There are some situations in which immediate breastfeeding is not possible or advisable. If your baby is premature, ill, in fragile condition, or if you are still struggling to recover from medication given for a cesarean section or any other type of sedation, you may need to postpone nursing. (For special issues such as cesarean sections, premature birth, and illness, sees Chapter 5.) If this is the case, there is still plenty of time to become acquainted with your baby. As soon as possible after a difficult delivery, request help from the hospital staff so that breastfeeding can go as smoothly as possible.

GETTING TO KNOW YOU: EARLY FEEDINGS

For many new moms, the first hours after your baby's birth will go by in a foggy but exciting blur. At long last, you are finally making the physical connection with the baby you've been wondering about for so many months. While most mothers and newborns prefer to rest for a few hours following an initial feeding, the time to practice nursing will soon follow. In order to avoid difficulties later, it is important to begin mastering the basics: how to position yourself, how to hold your baby, and how to make sure she's properly latched on. By practicing correct breastfeeding technique while you're in the hospital and have immediate access to expert help and support, you and your baby can get off to the best possible start.

∽   POSITIONS FOR BREASTFEEDING

Once you and your baby have become pros at breastfeeding, you'll be able to nurse while talking on the phone, reading a book, supervising your other children, or walking around. For now, though,

A Great Beginning

EARLY BREASTFEEDING BASICS

- Keep the baby skin to skin on your chest or abdomen right after delivery, and start breastfeeding within an hour of birth.

- Request that your baby not be fed any formula, water, or sugar water without a medical reason. Water and sugar water are generally not needed. Do not allow your newborn to be given a pacifier. If your baby wants to suck, you are encouraged to breastfeed her. Ask your obstetrician or pediatrician to write an order about this if needed.

- Keep your newborn with you day and night.

- Breastfeed on demand as soon as your baby shows hunger cues such as increased alertness or activity, smacking her lips, making suckling motions, or rooting (moving her head around in search of your breast). Don't wait until your baby begins to cry, which is a late sign of hunger. Feed for as long as your baby desires, until she detaches spontaneously from each breast.

- Alternate the breast you offer first at each feeding to ensure equal breast stimulation and milk removal. This improves your milk supply. Offer the second breast if your baby still seems hungry after feeding from one breast. Older babies will tend to feed from both breasts at each feeding. Young infants may be satisfied with one breast.

- Shortly after delivery, and again prior to discharge, have a lactation specialist, a nurse experienced in breastfeeding, or your doctor monitor your nursing technique to be sure everything is going well. Request a follow-up evaluation with your pediatrician within twenty-four to seventy-two hours after

leaving the hospital (or by the time your baby is three to five
days old).

- If you must be separated from your baby and cannot
breastfeed directly, express your milk for your baby.
(Ask a nurse or lactation specialist for help expressing
milk.)

it's best to start with as few distractions as possible. Most new
mothers first try breastfeeding sitting up in a hospital bed, with the
baby supported by a pillow in their lap and cradled in their arms.
If you choose this position, elevate the head of the bed as much as
possible and place pillows behind you until your back is comfortable. Place your baby on a pillow on your lap (this is an especially
good idea if you've given birth by cesarean section, or C-section) so
his head is level with your breast. You might put pillows at your
sides to rest your arms on so they won't tire in mid-feeding. At
home, you may find an armchair helpful. If you breastfeed while
sitting in a chair, be sure it offers sturdy back and arm support and
is not too low or high. A pillow or two tucked behind your back
can make nursing in a chair more comfortable, as can a low footstool to support your legs. It is always important to make sure that
you are comfortable before beginning the feeding.

Whether you are sitting up in bed or have settled into an armchair, keep your back straight but relaxed as you offer your baby
the breast. Your baby may find it more difficult to latch on properly if you are leaning forward or back, since this changes the angle
at which he receives the breast; your back may soon feel the strain
of this as well. If your breasts are large, you might want to place a
rolled-up towel or receiving blanket beneath your breast to keep

your baby's mouth at a straight-on angle with the nipple, in addition to supporting the breast with your hand.

Once you are comfortably positioned, you can hold your baby in a number of ways. As you practice breastfeeding before leaving the hospital, try several positions (for both your baby and yourself) and ask your nurse or lactation specialist to check your technique. Using more than one position can help prevent nipple soreness and clogging of milk ducts, since different positions drain different areas of the breast more effectively. (For information on clogged milk ducts, see Chapter 8.) Some positions also work better than others in certain circumstances.

All of the positions described are for guidance only. There is not an absolute right or wrong way to hold your baby for breastfeeding. Every mother and baby find the positions that work well for them. If you are a first-time breastfeeding mother, however, you may find the following guidance helpful for getting started.

∞   THE CRADLE HOLD

The traditional position is called the *cradle hold* or *Madonna hold*. For this position, support your baby on the arm that's on the same

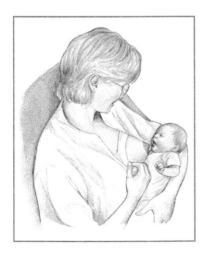

The cradle hold is the traditional breastfeeding position.

side as the breast you intend to use. Holding your upper arm close to your body, rest your baby's head in the crook of your elbow, support his back with your forearm, and cup his bottom or upper thigh with your hand. His arm may be positioned around your body or tucked slightly under his body to keep it out of the way. Once he's properly supported, rotate your forearm so his entire body turns toward you. His pelvis should be up against your abdomen, his chest against your chest, and his mouth lined up with your nipple. You can now bring your baby's mouth to the nipple (rather than the nipple to his mouth) without making him turn his head to the side. It is important for your baby's head to be aligned with the rest of his body instead of turned off to the side.

∞   THE CROSS-CRADLE HOLD

A variation on the cradle hold, the *cross-cradle* or *crossover hold* involves the same positioning except you support your baby on the arm opposite the breast being used. In this position, your hand supports your baby's neck and upper back, rather than his bottom, and his bottom rests either in the crook of your arm or on the pil-

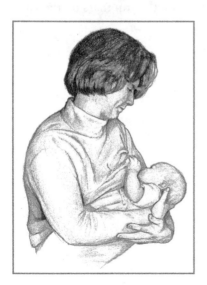

The cross-cradle hold is a good position for a young baby, because it provides good support for the baby's back.

low on your lap. Again, rotate your baby's body so it faces you and his mouth is lined up with your nipple. This is a good position for a baby who has difficulty latching on, because you can more easily guide his head into a better position by holding the back of his neck between your thumb and fingers.

☞ THE CLUTCH HOLD

Many breastfeeding women find that the *clutch hold,* also known as the *football hold,* is an easier position to maintain, particularly for those who have given birth by cesarean delivery, because it keeps the baby's weight off the abdominal incision. The clutch hold may also be useful for mothers of twins since one baby can nurse on each side, for women with large breasts or flat nipples since the mother can see both her nipple and her baby's mouth and can eas-

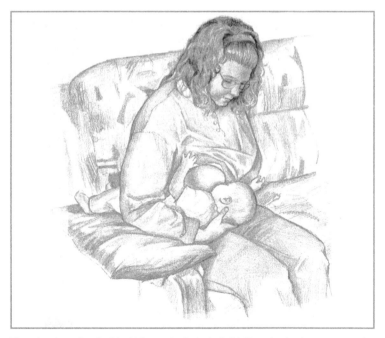

The clutch or football hold is particularly helpful if you've had a cesarean delivery because it keeps the baby's weight off the incision.

ily control the baby's head, and also for premature babies. In a clutch hold, your baby is held similarly to how you would hold a handbag clutched under your arm or a football clutched close to your body. To feed your baby in this position, place him beside you—on the side of the breast you will use—with his head near your breast. Tuck his body up against your side, under your arm. Your forearm should support his upper back, and your hand and fingers should support his shoulders, neck, and head. His legs will stretch out straight behind you or, if you are in a chair, you can rest his bottom against the back of the chair and angle his legs straight up. Finally, placing a pillow under your elbow for support, keep your baby's head level with your breast.

∽   RECLINING OR LYING DOWN

You may find that feeding your baby in a *reclining* position, rather than sitting, allows for some welcome relaxation. Nursing while lying down helps particularly if you have had a cesarean delivery or otherwise feel tired or unwell in the days following childbirth. To do this, lie on your side with one or more pillows behind your back

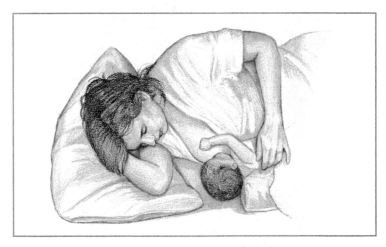

Feeding your baby in a reclining position lets you relax if you've had a cesarean delivery or feel tired in the days following childbirth.

and under your head for support. (A pillow placed between your knees may make you more comfortable.) Keep your back and hips in as straight a line as possible. Hold your baby closely on his side so he faces you with his mouth with your arm around him. Support your breast with your other hand while guiding your baby closer with the arm supporting him.

An advantage of this position is you don't have to get up to reposition your baby on your other breast. Simply place a pillow under him to elevate him until he's parallel with your upper breast and lean over farther to bring the upper breast to him. Or, if you prefer, hug him to your chest, roll over to your other side, and reposition him. You can support your baby by placing a pillow or rolled-up blanket behind his back, thus giving your lower arm a rest.

⊂⊃   ENSURING PROPER LATCH-ON

In any of the nursing positions described, when the baby is well aligned you should be able to draw a straight line that connects the baby's ear, shoulder, and hip on either side of the baby's body.

Once you and your baby are in proper position, the next step is to guide him toward the breast so that he can latch on properly and nurse. Latching on effectively is crucial to breastfeeding successfully because it prevents sore nipples, ensures sufficient milk supply, and stimulates plentiful milk production. In most cases (other than in the reclining position), it will be necessary to support your breast, at least in the early days of breastfeeding, in order for your baby to attach properly. This is especially true as milk production increases your breasts' size and weight. Using your free hand, place four fingers under your breast and your thumb on top to present the nipple to your baby. (Your lactation specialist or nurse may refer to this as a *C-hold,* since your hand makes the shape of a letter C.) Make sure your fingers are well behind the areola (the darker-colored area around the nipple) so it doesn't get in the way of your baby's latching on to the breast. You can provide

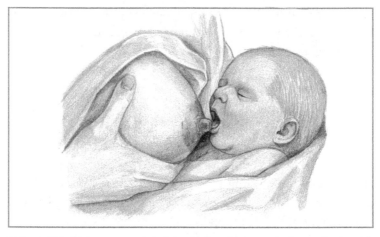

Using a C-hold, touch your baby's lower lip with your nipple to stimulate his rooting reflex.

gentle compression of the breast with your fingers to make it easier for your baby to latch. Alternatively, you can place your fingers on your breast in a scissors or V-hold to guide the nipple, but only if your fingers are wide enough apart to expose the areola.

With the breast supported, stroke your baby's lower lip with your nipple or bring his chin in to touch the breast closely. This causes him to open his mouth. (If his mouth stays closed, stroke his lip again, press gently down on his chin with your index finger, and open your own mouth, too, since he might imitate you.) When he opens wide—not just a little, but as though he's giving a big yawn—quickly draw him closer and place his open mouth fully on your breast. This guiding movement should be quick but gentle. Remember that you should bring your baby to your breast, not push your breast into his mouth. If your baby's head is pushed into the breast so hard that he cannot breathe, he may become agitated or frightened; he may arch his back and refuse to breastfeed.

If your baby is in proper nursing position, his jaws will come

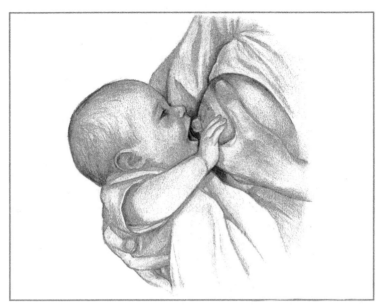

When your baby's mouth is wide open, bring him quickly but gently toward your breast.

together on your areola and his lips will seal over your breast. His chin and possibly his nose will touch your breast. (He will be able to breathe, but if you are concerned about his breathing, try lifting your breast or changing the angle of his body slightly, pulling his bottom in more closely to your body.) Helping him to latch on in a slightly asymmetric fashion, so that a bit more of the areola is in his mouth on the lower-lip side and a bit less on the upper-lip side, will position the nipple so it points toward the roof of the baby's mouth. You may feel slight discomfort when he first latches on and perhaps even for the first few sucks, but once he begins to suckle steadily you should not feel pain. *Pain beyond the first minute or so of nursing is a sign of improper latching on and should be immediately corrected through further practice or with the help of a pediatrician, family physician, nurse, or lactation specialist. When pain persists throughout nursing, detach the baby by inserting your finger in the corner of his mouth to break the suction and relatch him, making sure that his mouth is wide open before latching.*

Many new mothers assume that infants are born knowing instinctively how to attach themselves to the breast and that if you present your breast in the proper way he will know what to do. Certainly some babies are capable of self-attachment, with good technique. This is most likely to occur in the first hour after birth but can be repeated later on. (Researchers have studied infants who are able to maneuver themselves from the mother's lower abdomen, where they were placed immediately after delivery, up to the nipple, where they self-attach and start suckling. This has been called the "breast crawl." Videos of this are available on the Internet.)

Most newborns do easily learn to latch on to the breast and soon begin the deep, regular suckling and rhythmic swallowing that typify successful nursing. But not all babies know instinctively how to latch on. You may need to teach your baby until he experiences enough successful feedings to associate his feeding behaviors with the satiation of his hunger.

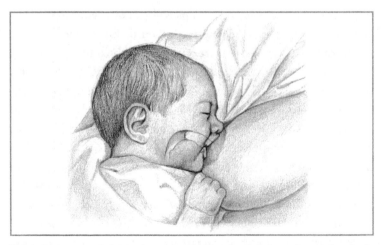

This baby is properly latched on when his lips cover the areola and the nipple is well inside his mouth, as you can see by this cross-sectional look inside the baby's mouth.

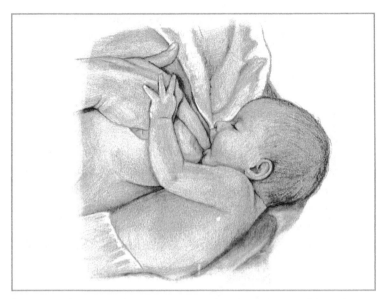

Sliding your finger between the baby's mouth and your breast releases the suction and detaches the baby comfortably, helping you avoid nipple pain.

The key to successful latching on involves taking enough of the breast into the mouth so that the nipple is drawn to the back of the baby's mouth and his gums and tongue are compressing the areola, covering about an inch or two of the areola from the base of the nipple. This suckling movement causes your baby's jaw to move the milk from the breast while his tongue makes a wavelike motion underneath the nipple, causing your milk to flow out through the tiny holes in your nipple. To achieve this, your baby's mouth must truly be open wide as he latches on. Many early nursing mistakes occur when the mother hasn't waited until her baby's jaws are about as wide as they can be before she pulls him to her breast. As a result, the baby sucks on the nipple only, a position that limits the amount of milk received and soon makes the nipple sore.

To help your baby take in a large mouthful, use your C-hold to gently compress your breast; this makes the areola narrower and the nipple stick out more so it is easier to grasp. As he latches on, his tongue should stick out a bit, cover his lower gum, and partially envelop the breast. His lips should turn outward and press against your breast.

If your infant doesn't manage to latch on properly the first time, gently detach him by sliding your finger into his mouth and pressing down on your breast to break the suction. You'll know your baby didn't latch on properly if you see indentations in his cheeks when he suckles, hear clicking noises, or notice his lips curled inward. He may also move his head frequently or not do any swallowing. Incorrect latching may also cause pain for you. Don't try to just pull him off your breast, since this could cause nipple pain. Keep practicing this latch-on technique until you and your newborn have mastered it, and don't hesitate to ask the hospital nurses and lactation specialists for help.

∞   BREASTFEEDING WITH INVERTED OR FLAT NIPPLES

As mentioned in Chapter 3, your baby may have a more difficult time latching on if your nipples are inverted or flat. Flat nipples may be almost indistinguishable from the areola, or protrude only slightly with stimulation. Inverted nipples retract inward, rather than becoming erect, when the areola is compressed. They may simply have a slight dimple in the center or may recede completely instead of protruding. (See illustrations on pages 37 and 38.) If your nipples are only mildly flat, your baby may be able to attach himself to the breast without any special help. If not, try gently compressing the areola to make the nipple as erect as possible before offering it to your infant.

If this doesn't help and you continue to have latch problems, it is important to get help from a skilled pediatrician, nurse, lactation specialist, or La Leche League volunteer as soon as possible. Your newborn's inability to latch on will lead to a decrease in milk supply if allowed to continue for more than a few days, and may increase the chance that your baby could become dehydrated. Continuing to try latching on without correcting the inversion can cause painful cracks in the nipples that will make breastfeeding more uncomfortable. A lactation specialist will monitor your baby's progress, help you gain access to any necessary equipment, show you how to supplement your baby's feedings with your own expressed milk when necessary, and assist you in correcting the problem as quickly and painlessly as possible. To draw your nipples out before breastfeeding, she may suggest using a hospital-grade electric breast pump or a manual pump, or possibly breast shells—plastic cups that press against the breast to help expose the nipples. In certain cases of flat nipples, a nipple shield, a thin silicone device that covers the breast and nipple, may be helpful in getting the baby properly latched in the first few days.

With a specialist's assistance, your baby should soon manage to attach to the breast properly and begin to breastfeed well. This process may take from one day to several weeks—not so long compared to the year or more you hope to nurse. Some persistent cases of inverted or flat nipples may need to be addressed by a knowledgeable physician. Occasionally some women have a severely inverted nipple on one side only and can nurse the baby on the other side. The mother will produce enough milk for her baby from only one breast, although over time, as she stops producing milk in the other breast, there will be a noticeable, but temporary, difference in the size of her breasts. If the baby does not breastfeed from one breast and the mother would like to protect the milk supply on that side, she can express her breast milk (using her hand or with a breast pump).

REFUSAL TO BREASTFEED

If your baby continues to have a problem latching on and you don't have inverted nipples, or if he outright refuses to breastfeed almost from birth, please get help from your pediatrician or lactation specialist immediately. A baby may be unable to latch on and suckle effectively during the early feedings due to the stress of labor and delivery or medications that were given during the birth process. It's also possible that your infant's natural temperament may cause him to resist being closely held and remaining calm enough to nurse. Be careful not to hold the top of your baby's head while breastfeeding because some babies pull away from the breast when pressure is applied to the back of their heads. In most cases— with the help of your lactation specialist, some patience, and a willingness to experiment—you will find a technique that satisfies both you and your newborn. On rare occasions there may be a condition in which the membrane connecting the tongue to the floor of the mouth is too tight. Your baby's pediatrician may be able to identify whether your baby has a problem with his mouth or oral structures, or with his nervous system, which interferes with successful latching and effective suckling.

∞ HICCUPS, SPIT-UPS, AND BURPS

You can tell that your baby has finished nursing from one breast when he has stopped suckling, fallen asleep, or drifted off the breast. If he's not asleep, he should seem calm and relaxed. Once he's finished, you can try to burp him to expel any air he has swallowed. Breastfed babies usually swallow less air than bottle-fed infants, so he may not need to burp. Burping may ease any feeling of fullness and may wake him up a bit so that you can offer him the other breast.

Almost all babies hiccup from time to time—a phenomenon that usually will bother you more than your infant but may distress him if he is in the middle of a feeding. As your milk supply increases, your baby may also spit up milk from time to time. This normal behavior is no cause for concern, but spit-ups and hiccups can be minimized by keeping your nursing sessions quiet and calm and changing your baby's position to help him relax.

If you choose to burp your baby after he finishes nursing on one side, hold him vertically against your body with his head over your shoulder. Place a clean cloth under his head to catch any spit-up and then *gently* pat or rub his back. If you prefer, you can perform this movement while sitting him on your lap and supporting his head with one hand or laying him across your knees on his stomach. If he hasn't burped after a few minutes, you can put him down to sleep on his back or offer him the other breast.

ᢒ LEARNING BY DOING

Like learning to ride a bicycle, type on a keyboard, or drive a car, it's easier to learn proper breastfeeding technique by doing it than by reading about it. Don't be put off if your first attempts are somewhat awkward. Remember, you and your baby are still tired from childbirth, and you, at least, are likely to feel emotionally overwhelmed. You may feel slightly uncomfortable at first with the physical sensation of breastfeeding, though that will pass. Some women feel some abdominal cramping during the first week or so of breastfeeding. This sensation, called *afterpains,* results from the release of the hormone oxytocin, which causes your uterus to shrink back to normal size and also helps your milk flow.

The fact that your breasts are producing only small quantities of colostrum at this point is also perfectly normal. Keep in mind that your milk volume will increase between two and five days after birth and that babies are designed to handle this. As we pointed out in Chapter 2, newborns usually lose some weight in the days immediately after birth, only to gain it back again shortly after the mother's milk supply increases. In the meantime, remember that what may seem complex today will seem increasingly natural and simple to you as time progresses. By keeping your long-term breastfeeding goals in mind, you can more easily meet any potential challenges from these first feedings and start creating a healthy life for your baby.

SUPPLY AND DEMAND: ESTABLISHING A BREASTFEEDING RHYTHM

As natural as it is, breastfeeding can often be confusing to a new mom. The colostrum may not look as you expected. Your baby

A Breastfeeding Checklist:
How to Tell If You're Nursing Correctly

Signs of Correct Nursing
- Your baby's mouth is open wide with lips turned out.
- His chin and nose are resting against the breast.
- He has taken as much of the areola as possible into his mouth.
- He is suckling rhythmically and deeply, in short bursts separated by pauses.
- You can hear him swallowing regularly.
- Your nipple is comfortable after the first few suckles.

Signs of Incorrect Nursing
- Your baby's head is not in line with his body.
- He is sucking on the nipple only, instead of suckling on the areola with the nipple far back in his mouth.
- He is sucking in a light, quick, fluttery manner rather than taking deep, regular sucks.
- His cheeks are puckered inward or you hear clicking noises.
- You don't hear him swallow regularly after your milk production has increased.
- You experience pain throughout the feed or have signs of nipple damage (such as cracking or bleeding).

may fall asleep before he gets anything to eat. Your breasts may become so engorged that they hurt. You may start to wonder if you'll ever establish a good breastfeeding rhythm with your baby.

In reality, the efficient supply-and-demand rhythm of normal breastfeeding—in which your baby's increased demand for milk spurs greater milk production from you and her diminished suckling decreases your milk supply—nearly always takes a while to establish fully and requires readjustment as your baby grows.

As your baby's suckling time increases, milk production will also increase. Her suckling stimulates nerve endings in your breast, sending a message to your brain that results in the release of the hormone prolactin. This plays a major role in stimulating milk to be created in your breasts using substances obtained from your bloodstream. While she breastfeeds, your prolactin levels surge, ensuring continued production of milk. If breastfeeding is decreased—if your infant is fed on a restricted schedule or given supplemental formula, water, sugar water, or even a pacifier to satisfy her suckling urge—your milk production will decrease accordingly.

Continued milk production depends not only on how much your baby suckles but also on how much milk she actually removes from your breast. If you were to breastfeed from only one breast, for example, the other breast would stop producing milk even though the hormones stimulated by nursing affect both breasts. This is one reason it's a good idea to alternate which breast you use to begin nursing. A baby who takes only the nipple into her mouth, or who otherwise attaches incorrectly and doesn't remove much milk, doesn't stimulate that breast to continue producing an adequate supply of milk. In fact, the protein contained in the residual milk remaining in the breast actually suppresses further milk production. To prevent this from happening, it's important to feed frequently from the very beginning.

The small early feedings are important to stimulate the greater milk production your baby will require in a few days' time. Newborns are born with extra water in their bodies, and weight loss normally occurs in the early days as the baby gets rid of this extra water, so they do not need much additional fluid. As your baby's need for fluid increases, a few days after delivery, your milk will increase in water (or fluid) content, and the composition of your milk will change. Over the next week or so, the protein content will decline and the fat and lactose content increase as your milk

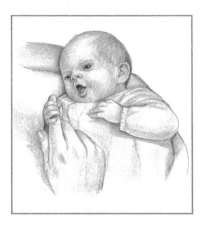

A baby's smacking lips and increased alertness and activity are
early signs of hunger.

gradually changes color from yellow to creamy white. By ten days
to two weeks after childbirth, your body will have begun producing fully mature milk, in even greater abundance than before. This
watery white or bluish milk contains all the nutrients your baby
needs and will increase and decrease in volume according to her
fluctuating demands.

Just as when learning to drive a car we sometimes push the ac-
celerator a little too hard and then not hard enough, it may take a
while for your body to adjust to your child's appetite changes.
Many mothers are surprised to see how little colostrum is available
initially and how much milk fills their breasts just a few days later.
This increase in milk production can lead to a tight, overfull feeling called *engorgement*. The solution to this problem is to feed your
infant frequently—eight to twelve times every twenty-four hours,
around the clock—even if you have to wake her to nurse. If she
sleeps for stretches of longer than four hours in the first two weeks,
wake her for a feeding. If she continues to sleep this long at a
stretch, repeatedly falls asleep soon after starting to breastfeed, or
seems listless or has a weak cry, inform her pediatrician right away.
Don't wait until your baby cries to feed her; keep an eye out for
early hunger cues such as smacking of lips, sucking on her hands,

and increased activity. You may also need to express some milk by hand or with a pump to ease your discomfort and to soften the nipple and areola enough so that the baby can latch on.

Eventually (usually quite soon), your milk production will adjust to the level your infant currently requires. During periods when she feeds more frequently—usually in response to growth spurts—your milk production will increase. (Growth spurts most commonly occur at approximately three weeks, six weeks, three months, and six months of age, but this varies from baby to baby.) Your milk supply will decrease again when her feeding sessions decrease. You will become expert at having her suckle a little longer or more frequently when you are concerned that you may not be producing enough milk and adding a few brief "topping-off" feedings on those days when you feel somewhat engorged. This ability to tailor your milk production to both her and your needs is one of the marvels of breastfeeding.

Q & A

Is Everything Okay?

Q: *I know several women who wanted to breastfeed but had to switch to formula because they didn't have enough milk. Could this happen to me?*

A: It is rarely necessary to switch to formula because a woman is *unable* to produce enough milk for her baby. Nearly all women can breastfeed successfully, assuming they receive enough support and information. The women you know who didn't have enough milk probably did not breastfeed frequently or long enough or did not manage to get their babies latched on to the breast properly. If their babies were given supplemental feedings or a pacifier, their infants'

subsequent nursing efforts may not have been adequate to stimulate enough milk production.

The volume of human milk naturally fluctuates quite a bit during the first two or three weeks. The best initial solution when a
newborn cries for a feeding or wakes frequently in the night to
breastfeed is to continue nursing as often as possible to stimulate
milk production. By using good breastfeeding techniques and focusing on exclusive breastfeeding, you will find that your baby's demand will increase your milk supply. The early days and weeks are
crucial in terms of getting breastfeeding off to a good start.

Q: *I was so involved in getting to know my baby and learning to
breastfeed in the days following childbirth, I felt like the baby's father did
not have much to do. He was as excited about our child's arrival as I
was. Is there some way to involve the father in the early breastfeeding
process?*

A: Just as your baby's father supported you through the birthing
process, he can act as an effective coach through the early stages of
breastfeeding (see Chapter 11 for more on the father's role). By remaining present when you meet with physicians, nurses, and lactation specialists, and by referring to this book, he can help you
position your baby correctly when learning to nurse. He can keep
an eye on the latching-on process, making sure your infant is in the
proper position for getting milk. He can arrange pillows to better
support your back during feeding sessions and hold and cuddle the
baby when you need a rest. He may tickle your baby's foot or rub
her back during a feeding to keep her stimulated if she starts to fall
asleep. Or he can help burp the baby. If you gave birth by cesarean
delivery, you will be especially grateful for his help as you gradually
recuperate from surgery. Certainly he can play an important role
by changing your baby's diapers, dressing her, playing with her, and
giving her baths. By encouraging him to help nurture your baby in

these valuable ways, you will include him in the process of helping your newborn attach in a unique way to each of her parents.

Q: *I find that breastfeeding hurts a lot for the minute or so after my baby latches on. I know how important human milk is for her, but the initial pain makes me want to give up. Will this situation change?*

A: Some new mothers feel more discomfort than others during different aspects of the breastfeeding process, and some women have nipples that are naturally more sensitive. Some feel, as you do, that the first few suckles of a breastfeeding session are uncomfortable, especially in the early weeks. This is referred to as "latch-on pain." It may help to know that most of these sensations fade after the first couple of weeks of breastfeeding. Other mothers dislike the feeling they experience as their milk lets down, but most mothers readily adjust to this brief pins-and-needles sensation. If this discomfort is mild and brief, reassess how you feel in a few weeks. If you have severe pain or discomfort that does not diminish as the baby settles into nursing, ask for help with latching on and request pain medication, if needed, that's safe to take when breastfeeding. You need a licensed experienced certified lactation consultant to help you if you experience severe discomfort. This is not normal and indicates a problem that needs to be corrected as soon as possible to ensure breastfeeding success.

HOW OFTEN TO BREASTFEED

"How often should I feed my baby?" is one of the most frequent questions new mothers ask. For the reasons outlined in the previous section, the simple answer to that question is "As often as he's willing." Don't wait until your baby cries to put him to the breast.

Crying is a late sign of hunger. He will indicate his desire to breast-feed long before he cries by smacking his lips, making suckling motions, rooting (moving his head around in search of your breast), kicking and squirming, or looking more alert. Your baby may give you such signals as often as every hour or so in the early days after birth. He should not go longer than about two to three hours during the day or three to four hours at night without a feeding. Even

Is My Newborn Getting Enough Milk?

Nearly all new mothers worry about whether their babies are properly nourished. Breastfeeding mothers cannot measure exactly how much milk their newborns take, but they can tell in other ways whether their babies are getting enough to eat. Your well-nourished newborn should:

- Lose no more than 7 percent of his birthweight in the first few days after birth before starting to gain weight again.
- Have one or two bowel movements per day on days one and two, with blackish, tarry stools, and at least two stools that are beginning to appear greenish to yellow on days three and four. By five to seven days, his stools should be yellow and loose, with small curds, and should number at least three to four per day. When your milk production increases, your baby will often stool with each feeding for the first month of life.
- Have six or more wet diapers per day, with nearly colorless or pale yellow urine, by five to seven days.
- Seem satisfied and happy for an average of one to three hours between feedings.
- Nurse at least eight to twelve times every twenty-four hours.

if you have to wake him up, be sure he receives eight to twelve feedings in every twenty-four-hour period. If he does not feed at first upon being awakened, wait half an hour, wake him up, and try again. Some babies will nurse even when they are not wide awake, so you don't have to awaken them completely.

Soon you will become familiar with your baby's feeding style—active and eager, sleepy and dreamy, or focused and intent. In the meantime, encourage him to feed as long as possible at each feeding. Keep him at your breast as long as he is actively suckling. Detaching a suckling baby from your breast before he's finished, or allowing him to fall asleep shortly after beginning to feed, may throw off the breastfeeding rhythm of supply and demand. Allow him to breastfeed until he seems full (at this point he will probably detach from the breast all by himself). Keep in mind that the longer your baby nurses, the higher the fat content of the milk he is drinking. This higher-fat milk will help him to grow well and make him more satisfied between feedings. If he begins to drift off to sleep after nursing for only a few minutes, try rubbing his back or gently tickling his feet to keep him awake enough to breastfeed a little while longer. Shorter, timed nursing periods may not allow him the opportunity to enjoy the full benefits of your milk and may leave your breasts full of unreleased milk, making you feel engorged and uncomfortable.

COPING WITH JAUNDICE

Many infants develop jaundice within several days after birth. A baby becomes jaundiced when bilirubin, which is produced naturally by the body as a by-product of red blood cells, builds up faster than a newborn's liver can break it down and get rid of it in the baby's stool. Too much bilirubin makes a baby's skin and eyes look yellow. Since drinking human milk helps remove bilirubin through the baby's stools, babies who are not breastfeeding adequately are at greater risk of developing jaundice. Jaundice usually resolves on its

Knowledge Is Power

EDUCATING YOURSELF

Unless you delivered via cesarean section or are facing some other complications relating to childbirth, your time in the hospital is likely to be quite brief and full of so many new experiences that you may feel overwhelmed by the time you pack to go home. Nevertheless, your hospital stay represents one of your best chances to learn more about breastfeeding while you have help available twenty-four hours a day. Take an active role in your breastfeeding education. Make sure you request help from your physician, nurse, or lactation specialist the first time the baby breastfeeds. After that, continue to practice until you feel comfortable nursing. Before leaving the hospital, ask the nurse to observe your breastfeeding technique and answer the questions you have. Limiting the number of hospital visitors may give you more opportunity to feel comfortable with breastfeeding while you do have plenty of support. Most hospitals offer breastfeeding classes for new mothers, which are well worth attending; some provide videos on breastfeeding and other aspects of newborn care in the hospital or offer in-house television programs. In addition, the La Leche League is a phone call away. Talking with other breastfeeding mothers may provide just the information or morale boost you need. If you do not feel you're receiving the support you need from hospital staff during the days following childbirth, tell your pediatrician or nurse, and ask for help from a lactation specialist.

own, but more serious cases may require treatment with special lights that help break down the bilirubin and allow it to be cleared from the baby's system. Feeding more frequently or for longer periods of time to help pass the bilirubin in the stools is almost always helpful. Certainly there is no reason to stop breastfeeding if your baby develops jaundice of this type. In select cases of jaundice, your pediatrician might recommend a formula supplement as a temporary measure.

Occasionally jaundice lasts longer than two weeks. You can still usually continue breastfeeding. Rarely your pediatrician may ask you to stop breastfeeding for a day or two. If you must interrupt breastfeeding for any reason, be sure to express your milk using a quality electric breast pump (see Chapter 5) so you can keep producing milk and can restart nursing easily. Your nurse, lactation specialist, or La Leche League group can give you guidance in using a breast pump.

A NEW LIFE

By the time you leave the hospital, which is typically a matter of days, you should have at least some idea of how to breastfeed your new baby. You may even have experienceed great success. You should have had a visit from your pediatrician—or another health care professional—who will check on your breastfeeding technique and offer suggestions. And if you've prepared yourself physically and emotionally for the road ahead, you'll have laid the groundwork that will support your decision to breastfeed once you get home. For you and your baby, this will mark the start of a unique relationship, one that will benefit your infant for years to come.

CHAPTER 5

Special Situations

Every mother naturally hopes for a normal vaginal birth without any complications, but sometimes things don't work out that way. You may go into labor early and have a premature baby. Your infant may be born with an illness you didn't anticipate. Your baby may be born unexpectedly by cesarean delivery. Or you might have health problems that make you wonder if breastfeeding is even an option.

Special birth situations may introduce challenges into the typical breastfeeding process. The best way to deal with such challenges—and other situations that arise weeks or even months later—is to be knowledgeable about the solutions available, stay in close contact with your pediatrician, maintain a reliable and educated support network to help you in times of need, and simply make the decision to breastfeed through rough times as well as easy ones.

SPECIAL BIRTHS

Your birthing experience may affect the way you initiate breastfeeding in a number of ways. Contrary to your expectations, you may have been given anesthesia during childbirth, or your baby may have been born with a condition that makes nursing difficult. As challenging as you may find it to initiate breastfeeding under these conditions, remember that you have the advantage of well-informed breastfeeding specialists ready to assist you. It may help to know that no matter what the situation, mothers in similar circumstances have been able to breastfeed successfully.

∞ CESAREAN DELIVERY

A common circumstance is a cesarean delivery, often referred to as a C-section, instead of a vaginal birth. If the C-section is done without prior planning, you may have endured a long and difficult delivery. If that's the case, your doctor may be more worried about your rest and recovery and less likely to encourage you to breastfeed right after delivery. You may also feel disappointed by this unexpected turn of events, which may inhibit the let-down and flow of your breast milk. Women who have planned C-sections, on the other hand, often know what to expect and are fully prepared to breastfeed their newborn.

The good news is that the method of delivery has little effect on your ability to nurse your baby. Your breast milk will come in almost as readily as it would have if you had delivered vaginally. It is especially important to begin breastfeeding as soon as you are able and to continue breastfeeding your baby on a frequent basis to ensure a good milk supply. Even if you need a few hours to recover from your surgery, you will be able to breastfeed as soon as you feel up to it.

Most drugs administered to mothers who give birth by cesarean delivery do not seriously affect the infant. You will probably receive a regional anesthetic, such as an epidural, rather than the general anesthesia that once made women unconscious during the delivery. Since less regional anesthesia gets into your bloodstream than with general anesthesia, it causes less sedation in the newborn. Some newborns tend to be a bit sleepy following an epidural and may suckle with less enthusiasm at first, but no long-term negative effects on full-term babies' development or ability to breastfeed have been demonstrated. Even if you are given general anesthesia, you should be able to breastfeed as soon as you're awake enough. When you are counseled about a cesarean delivery, it is a good idea to remind the obstetrician and anesthesiologist that you intend to breastfeed.

Following a cesarean delivery, your doctor will give you pain medications, initially through your IV and later in pill form, to help make you comfortable. In most cases, little of this medication passes through your breast milk to your baby. Some pain medications may temporarily make your newborn a little sleepy, but the benefits of breastfeeding far outweigh this potential drowsiness. Pain interferes with the release of oxytocin, a hormone which helps your milk to flow readily for your baby, so adequate control of your pain is important. If you have any concerns about the pain medication you are being offered, speak with your doctor or lactation specialist.

Your abdominal incision may make finding a comfortable breastfeeding position a little more difficult at first. You might adjust some of the basic positions by sitting up in bed, using one or two extra pillows to support your baby on your lap and protect your incision, by lying down on your side with your baby facing you, or by using a football hold with enough pillows to raise your baby's head to the level of the breast (see Chapter 4). Make sure to get into a comfortable position before beginning to breastfeed, and don't be shy about asking for help. As your incision heals and you are able to move about more readily, nursing will become much easier—but expect to need some extra rest and assistance until you are fully back on your feet again. Be grateful for the help of family and friends with household chores, so you can concentrate on recovery from surgery and breastfeeding your baby.

⌒ PREMATURE BIRTHS AND NEWBORN ILLNESS

Providing breast milk for a premature or seriously ill newborn may be a challenge, but it is usually possible and it is certainly an effective way to enhance your baby's health, growth, and development. Even if your baby is unable to breastfeed at first, you can begin expressing your milk immediately after giving birth. When she is stable, she can have the milk fed to her by a tube or by letting her sip the milk from a tiny cup or bottle. No matter how your breast milk is delivered to her, it provides the best nourishment possible at a time when such an advantage makes a big difference.

Mothers of premature babies produce breast milk that is slightly different in composition, at least for the first several weeks, and this difference is designed to meet your baby's particular needs. The premature milk is higher in protein and minerals, such as salt, and contains different types of fat that she can more easily digest and absorb. The fat in human milk helps to enhance the development of the baby's brain and neurologic tissues, which is especially important for premature infants. Human milk is easier for her to digest than formula and avoids exposing her immature intestinal lining to the cow's milk proteins found in premature infant formula. Prema-

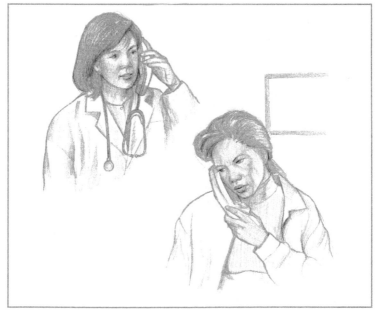

Ask your child's pediatrician or other members of your support team for any assistance you need while breastfeeding.

ture babies who are breastfed are less likely to develop intestinal infections than are babies who are formula-fed. The milk you produce in the first few days contains high concentrations of antibodies to help your baby fight infection. Even if your baby cannot breastfeed yet, expressing breast milk from the beginning will ensure that your milk supply is maintained until your baby is able to nurse.

Your first step in providing your baby with breast milk is to enlist the support of the medical personnel who will care for your infant at the hospital. Notify your baby's pediatrician and neonatologist, if one is caring for your baby, of your desire to breastfeed and to provide your expressed breast milk for your baby. Your doctors can arrange to have your expressed milk fed to your baby or for you to breastfeed your infant in the neonatal intensive care unit (NICU). Many hospitals now provide private areas for nursing and trained specialists to assist breastfeeding mothers. Ask your baby's nurse or a lactation consultant in the NICU for assistance. These experienced members of your support team can show you how to assemble and use an electric breast pump, teach you to express milk efficiently, and give you advice on storing breast milk (see Chapter 9). If you are able to directly breastfeed, they can help you adjust your nursing position to your infant's small size. Many neonatal intensive care units encourage parents to room in continuously and keep the baby skin to skin, sometimes referred to as kangaroo care, because this has been shown to be beneficial for stability and optimal growth and development of premature babies. Breast milk pumping, or expression, immediately after holding your baby skin to skin is a very effective way to increase your milk supply. Some mothers find pumping at their baby's bedside in the NICU very helpful as well.

If your newborn is too small or ill to breastfeed at first, or if a birth condition prevents her from breastfeeding directly, you will find that a hospital-grade electric breast pump is an effective way to express milk and establish and maintain an adequate milk supply. Your hospital will provide you with a pump while you are there, and you can rent or purchase one to use at home later. The pump you use should create a milking action and not simply be a sucking device. Beginning as soon as possible after your baby's birth, express your milk at regular intervals, at approximately the times when your baby would usually feed. Aim to pump at least six to eight times a day; this provides nipple stimulation and encourages milk production. You should pump at regular intervals throughout the night for the first few weeks, and not sleep for more than four or five hours at a time. If you wake up each morning and your breasts feel full, then you are sleeping too long through the night; this fullness will actually diminish your milk production. Using a double-pump setup lets you express milk from both breasts at the same time. Most women find that the double pump produces the most milk in the least amount of time. When using the pump, continue to pump for several minutes after your milk has stopped flowing to stimulate increased milk production. For mothers of preterm babies the minimum amount of time to try to pump throughout a twenty-four-hour period is one hundred minutes. This much breast stimulation and milk expression is the minimum required to maintain breast milk supply over many weeks (if your baby is very small, premature, or ill).

Breast massage before and during the use of the pump has been shown to improve your milk flow and may even boost your milk production. To do this, make small, circular motions with your fingertips, starting at the outer edges of your breast near the chest wall, and slowly make your way toward the center. The massage should always be gentle to avoid producing friction on the skin surface or massaging so deeply that it causes pain.

Keep in mind that you will express only small amounts of colostrum at first, but this immune-boosting substance is extremely beneficial for your baby. Some mothers find that expressing the colostrum by hand massage into a small cup or spoon is easier than using an electric pump in the first few days. Hand expression into a cup also allows you to save each drop, instead of los-

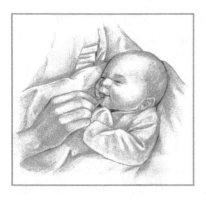

If your baby is born prematurely or with an illness, your expressed breast milk may be fed to her from a tiny cup, tube, or bottle.

ing milk that is trapped within the tubing of the pump. Once your milk supply increases, the amount of milk you can express will probably fluctuate from day to day. As a result, you will need to increase the number of times per day you express milk to maintain an optimal milk supply. These fluctuations are normal—just more easily observed when expressing milk than when breastfeeding. Once your baby begins breastfeeding, your milk production is likely to increase. To maximize your milk production, try to get as much rest as possible, take your prescribed pain medication, drink adequate fluids, and minimize stress.

Your breast milk can be fed to your baby through a tube that passes through her nose or mouth into her stomach or from a tiny cup or bottle. The feeding route will depend on the degree of prematurity of your infant and on the policies in the NICU at your hospital. Occasionally young infants fed by bottle may start to prefer the bottle, which delivers milk faster and with less effort than feeding at the breast. Some of these babies later refuse to breastfeed—a situation called *nipple confusion* or *nipple preference*. During this period when your baby is using an alternative feeding method, you can introduce her to breastfeeding by holding her skin to skin against your chest whenever possible and allowing her to nuzzle and suckle at your breast. This, of course, should be done only when the neonatologist or pediatrician has given approval.

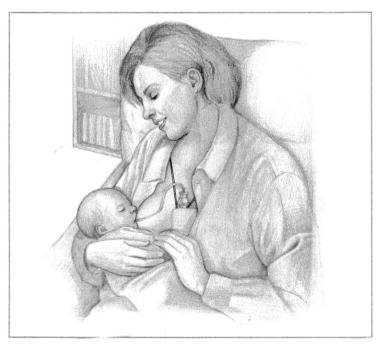

A nursing supplementer delivers milk through a tube taped next to the nipple.

Soon you may be able to progress to a nursing supplementer or other device that will deliver your expressed breast milk from a bottle or syringe through a tiny tube that is taped next to your nipple. With this method, your baby should begin to feed partly from the tube and partly from your breast as he latches on to your breast and actively nurses.

Early breastfeeding sessions will probably be more successful if you time them for when your baby is most awake and alert but calm. Experiment with different nursing positions (see Chapter 4) to discover which works best for the two of you. Mothers of preterm babies often find the cross-cradle hold to be the easiest to use while "teaching" their baby how to latch on. Even if your baby doesn't suckle at the breast, you can express some milk onto your nipple, so your baby tastes your breast milk when she comes into contact with the areola and nipple. A premature baby often tires rather easily, so these early feedings are likely to be brief. (You can use your remaining time together to hold, rock, sing to, and cuddle your newborn.) Try to breastfeed as often as possible and continue to express milk for feedings in your absence. Frequent nursing and milk expression, as well as regular skin-to-skin holding, will help maintain your milk supply. An increasing number of hospitals allow mothers to room in, or stay overnight with their babies, on the night or two prior to discharge from the NICU, enabling the mothers to start to learn their infants' round-the-clock hunger cues and breastfeeding rhythms as well as other aspects of infant care before going home. Such experience can ease the transition from hospital to home life for you and your baby.

You will naturally want to focus on making the transition from feeding your expressed breast milk to direct breastfeeding, but understand that your hospital's medical staff wants to make sure your infant receives adequate calories and nutrition before she goes home. To achieve adequate growth and strong bones with enough calcium being deposited in them, neonatologists may enrich the diet of tiny preterm babies by adding special supplemental nutrients to the mothers' breast milk, often in the form of commercially available milk fortifiers. Occasionally the doctors may decide to feed an infant with special formulas for premature babies, sometimes alternating the formula with your breast milk. Even if your baby is not getting feedings at all due to medical complications, continue to express your breast milk and freeze it for later use, thus maintaining your milk production. In your conversations with the baby's doctor, be sure to reinforce your desire to breastfeed when it's medically appropriate.

After your baby is home from the hospital, you may need to keep using your breast pump until your baby is exclusively breastfeeding (actually nursing) and growing well without the need for any supplemental bottles or formula. This lets you store breast milk for extra feedings and maintain an adequate milk supply, especially as your baby grows and his needs increase. Attempt to nurse whenever your baby shows an interest—even if it's every hour or hour and a half during the early weeks. If your premature baby is exclusively breastfed, your pediatrician should recommend a multivitamin and iron supplement. Finally, have your breastfeeding technique rechecked by your pediatrician or a lactation specialist shortly after your baby's homecoming.

Caring for and learning to breastfeed a premature or ill newborn is emotionally taxing for any new mother. It's a good idea to contact support groups in your area that specialize in your baby's condition. Other mothers are often the most valuable sources of information. Make sure, too, that your partner and other family members understand the enormous advantages of breastfeeding a preterm baby or an ill hospitalized newborn. The emotional and practical support of your loved ones will go a long way in helping you achieve your breastfeeding goals.

⟳ TWINS AND OTHER MULTIPLES

If you are the new mother of twins, triplets, or a larger number of multiples, you may worry about how you will manage to breastfeed them all. If you have twins, you can breastfeed them at the same time by holding one baby at each side in a football hold (see Chapter 4) or by cradling both infants in front of you with their bodies crossing each other. You may also feed one baby using a football hold and the other in a cradle position. You can experiment and find the positions that work best for you.

You may need to express breast milk as well as breastfeed, since multiples are frequently born prematurely and require special care. A hospital-grade electric breast pump will help maximize your milk supply until your babies have fully adjusted to breastfeeding and are gaining weight appropriately. Your lactation specialist, local Mothers of Twins club, or La Leche League can offer advice

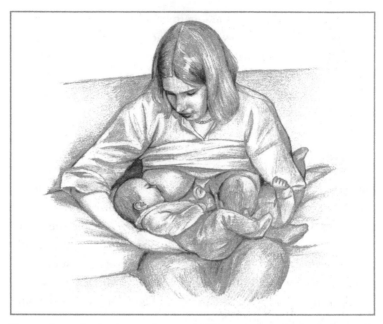

You can breastfeed twins simultaneously. This mother is using both the cradle hold and the football hold.

on where to find a pump and provide other helpful information. Your pediatrician will continue to monitor your babies' weights to make sure each is getting an adequate amount of breast milk to ensure proper weight gain.

If you have triplets, you can breastfeed them as well. But do not be discouraged if your pediatrician recommends supplementing feedings with formula. You might find nursing two of your babies at a time and giving formula or expressed breast milk to the third works the best. At the next feeding, give the formula to a different baby. All three (or more) babies should have a chance to breastfeed. And it's especially important for you to get adequate rest, eat a good diet, and have good help with household chores and baby care to establish and maintain a milk supply for all of your babies. One estimate found that breastfeeding twins may require an additional 1,500 extra calories a day!

CONSIDERING YOUR OWN HEALTH

For some new mothers, concerns about breastfeeding revolve less around their babies' physical condition than their own. Since some infectious diseases can be passed on to the baby through human milk, you will certainly want to discuss your medical history with your doctor and your baby's pediatrician. The American Academy of Pediatrics and the Centers for Disease Control and Prevention (CDC) advise mothers in the United States who are infected with HIV not to breastfeed, since the virus may be passed in the breast milk to their infant. They may, however, feed their babies pasteurized donor human milk if available. Donor milk is obtained from mothers who are free from HIV or other infectious diseases, and the milk is processed and pasteurized by a donor milk bank using standard procedures.

If you are infected with hepatitis B, your baby should receive the vaccination for hepatitis B—along with hepatitis B immune globulin (HBIG)—as soon as possible after birth. Giving these two injections soon after delivery is highly effective in preventing the spread of hepatitis B from mother to infant. In fact, the hepatitis B vaccine is recommended for all babies, whether their mother is infected with hepatitis B or not. Hepatitis B virus has been detected in human milk, but breastfeeding has not been shown to increase the risk of infection to the baby. The AAP states that maternal infection with hepatitis B is compatible with breastfeeding and there is no need to delay initiation of breastfeeding until the infant is immunized against hepatitis B.

Both the AAP and the CDC state that maternal infection with hepatitis C is also compatible with breastfeeding. Though an infant can be infected with hepatitis C during pregnancy or delivery, breastfed infants do not have higher rates of hepatitis C than formula-fed infants. Breastfeeding may even help prevent the spread of hepatitis C from the mother to the baby, by providing antibodies passed to the baby through the breast milk.

Other types of infections need to be evaluated by your obstetrician, pediatrician, or family physician, but few will prevent breastfeeding. This is true even when the infection or inflammation involves the breast itself—as in the case of mastitis, an infection of a section of the breast. This condition is typically treated with antibiotics, frequent breastfeeding, and/or expression of milk with a pump, adequate fluids, pain medication, and rest.

If you have tuberculosis (TB), you may breastfeed if you are currently taking medication. Mothers with untreated TB at the time of delivery should not breastfeed or be in direct contact with their newborn until they have started appropriate drug treatment and they are no longer infectious. In most cases, you can safely breastfeed after you have been taking antibiotics for about two weeks and have been told by your doctor that you are no longer infectious. You should begin pumping soon after delivery, and your pumped milk may be fed to your infant until you can breastfeed directly. If you have had a positive TB skin test but a normal chest X-ray, talk to your doctor to see if you need to be treated with any medication, but you can breastfeed in this circumstance.

∞   CANCER

If you have been diagnosed with breast cancer in the past and have been treated for it, you may be concerned about the effects of breastfeeding on you and your baby. Previous breast cancer does not mean that you cannot breastfeed your baby. If you have had a mastectomy, you can feed from the remaining breast. If you have had a tumor removed from your breast or radiation treatments, you can still try feeding from that breast. You may find that your milk production is less, however. Always discuss your breastfeeding options with your physician.

∞   BREAST SURGERY

In the past, there have been concerns about the safety of breastfeeding after breast enlargement with breast implants. But there is

What Is That?

DISCOVERING A LUMP WHILE BREASTFEEDING

Some women get plugged milk ducts, which are painful or sensitive to the touch but can be easily treated (see Chapter 8). And lactating breasts may feel lumpy. However, do not ignore a lump or bump in your breast that develops during lactation and does not go away with gentle massage and breastfeeding or milk expression. While less common in younger women, a lump may represent the first signs of breast cancer and must be evaluated by your physician. Mammograms are more difficult for a radiologist to interpret during lactation. Nevertheless, breast self-exams and annual physician breast exams should continue throughout the lactation period.

It is possible to continue breastfeeding while undergoing mammograms and other diagnostic procedures, including ultrasounds and biopsies, though a temporary interruption is sometimes necessary from that breast. If you have a lump or cyst removed, it is generally safe to breastfeed afterward. Monitor your baby's weight gain, however, as surgical incisions may sever milk ducts and nerves related to milk production and release.

no evidence that silicone breast implants cause any harm to the baby, and the newer saline (saltwater-filled) implant devices do not cause any problems, either. In most cases, plastic surgery to enlarge the breasts should not interfere significantly with your ability to breastfeed—provided the nipples have not been moved and no milk ducts have been cut. In certain cases of breast enlargement, the women had underdeveloped breast tissue, which was the reason that breast enlargement was undertaken. In these cases, the relative lack of breast glandular tissue may interfere with the production of adequate breast milk. With any previous breast surgery, the baby will need to be monitored carefully to make sure that he is getting enough milk.

Surgery to reduce the size of breasts (breast reduction) is more likely to interfere with breastfeeding, especially if the nipples were repositioned during the course of the surgery—resulting in the total cutting of milk ducts or nerves. Many women who have had this type of breast surgery are able to breastfeed, however, and the longer it has been since the surgery, the more likely that breastfeeding, or at least partial breastfeeding, will be successful.

If you have had any surgical procedure on your breast, even a biopsy, make sure that your baby's doctor knows this. By all means begin breastfeeding, making sure that your pediatrician or family physician closely monitors your infant to be certain that he is receiving adequate breast milk.

ROUTINE ILLNESSES

Even the healthiest mothers sometimes get sick. If you are temporarily unable to breastfeed because of a severe illness or while taking certain medications, keep up your milk supply by expressing milk either by hand, with a manual breast pump (see Chapter 9), or with an electric pump (see Chapter 10). Obviously, this process is not the same as actual breastfeeding, and it may seem pointless if the breast milk needs to be discarded while your baby receives previously expressed milk, donor breast milk, or formula. But remember that while your illness will not last long, breastfeeding may continue for months or years. By using a pump to maintain your milk production, you can ensure an ongoing breastfeeding relationship with your child after you recover and for a long time to come. In rare instances, when the mother is unable to pump because of severe illness, hospital staff can express milk to maintain comfort, decrease the risk of developing a breast infection, and ensure continued milk production. Fortunately, these more serious illnesses are rare, and more common simple infections rarely interfere with your ability to breastfeed your baby.

MEDICATIONS: WHAT TO TAKE, AND WHAT NOT TO TAKE, WHILE BREASTFEEDING

After delivery, many women are relieved that they no longer have to worry that taking a pain reliever or cold pill may negatively affect the development of their growing fetus. Still, if you are breastfeeding and plan to take any kind of drug—whether prescription or over-the-counter—be sure to get the approval of your obstetric or pediatric health care provider. Most medications are safe during breastfeeding, but a few can have serious side effects for your baby—and they are not necessarily the same ones that were most concerning during pregnancy. Your doctor is the best source of the most up-to-date information on which medications are safe for you at this time.

Much is still unknown regarding long-term effects of various kinds of medications. For this reason, it's important to take medication only when absolutely necessary while breastfeeding, to use the safest drug, and to take the lowest dose possible. When possible, use short-acting drugs rather than longer-acting varieties. Short-acting drugs are best taken immediately after a nursing session, while sustained-release medications should be taken just after your baby's last evening feeding or before his longest sleep period. When taking any medication, watch closely for reactions in your baby, including loss of appetite, diarrhea, sleepiness, excessive crying, vomiting, or skin rashes. Call your baby's pediatrician immediately if any of these symptoms appear. In the unlikely event that your doctor needs to prescribe a potentially harmful drug for a short time, you can express and store your milk ahead of time and then express and discard the milk with the drug until the medication is cleared from your body. The length of time required to clear the drug from your system varies based on the particular medication, but your doctor should advise you about this.

○♡ BIRTH CONTROL

Frequent, exclusive breastfeeding (no water, juice, formula, solid foods, or other supplements for the baby), including at least one

---

Home Cures

HOMEOPATHIC AND HERBAL MEDICINES

Many Americans are accustomed to turning to homeopathic remedies to treat routine illnesses, particularly when they are concerned about side effects associated with more mainstream medicines. However, just because a remedy is "natural" doesn't mean it's safe for breastfeeding women or their babies. In many cases, very little scientific research has been done regarding the implications of using such treatments while nursing. In the United States, the Food and Drug Administration (FDA) does not regulate homeopathic, herbal, or natural remedies, meaning that the government does not oversee these products for purity or to make sure there are no toxic substances. When taken in large quantities, certain substances create negative effects such as increased blood pressure and reduced milk supply. It's best to treat homeopathic remedies just as you would any medicine: Refrain from taking herbs or other homeopathic medications (aside from commercially produced herbal teas) unless your family physician, obstetrician, or pediatrician has approved them. Take approved substances in the smallest doses possible and carefully observe your baby for any negative reactions. Make sure your doctor and your baby's pediatrician are aware of anything you are taking.

---

night feeding, significantly reduces the chance of your becoming pregnant during the first six months after birth. However, after about six weeks, especially if you are only partially breastfeeding, you can begin using contraceptives if your milk supply is firmly established. You should discuss the issue with your obstetrician or gynecologist. While there are no harmful effects on infants when mothers use hormonal contraceptives, research has shown that birth control pills with high doses of estrogen may decrease milk supply. Progestin-only pills (sometimes referred to as mini-pills) are least likely to interfere with breastfeeding, although they have increased side effects for the mother. Effects vary from woman to woman and with the type of pill, so discuss the possible ramifications with your doctor before you begin taking contraceptives. You might also consider using condoms, a diaphragm, or a cervical cap and spermicide instead, since these forms of birth control are least likely to interfere with your milk supply.

CIGARETTES

Smoking cigarettes is not recommended for mothers who breastfeed. Nicotine, the addictive substance that you inhale when smoking cigarettes, passes through breast milk to your baby. Both nicotine and its by-product, cotinine, can be detected in the urine of babies whose mothers smoke, whether or not the mothers breastfeed, so some exposure comes from the breast milk and some from the environment. Nicotine can cause babies to be restless and jittery, eat poorly, and not sleep as well. Babies exposed to secondhand smoke can also be exposed to additional toxic substances, such as carbon monoxide and cyanide.

If you want to join a stop-smoking program or begin using nicotine patches or gum, discuss these plans with your doctor or pediatrician. Nicotine patches or gum should never be used by breastfeeding mothers who are still smoking. The baby may develop toxic or harmful levels of nicotine in his system. If you stop smoking and use nicotine patches or gum, your baby will be exposed only to nicotine and not to the other by-products of tobacco, so this is preferable.

If you find you're unable to quit and do continue to smoke, limit yourself to as few cigarettes a day as possible. Take your cigarette breaks immediately after a breastfeeding session.

It is also important to consider the effects of secondhand smoke on your baby. Inhaling smoke in this way has been shown to increase the risk of sudden infant death syndrome (SIDS) and is also related to an increased risk of respiratory illnesses such as coughs, asthma, and ear infection. To protect your baby from these effects, never smoke while holding or breastfeeding her, go outside your home to smoke, and never smoke in your car. Residual smoke remains in your hair and on your clothing after you have had a cigarette, so your baby continues to smell and inhale it.

∽   RECREATIONAL DRUGS

In no case are recreational drugs advisable for breastfeeding mothers, since the effect of these drugs on infants may be harmful, lasting, and, at the very least, highly unpredictable. Studies have shown that SIDS is more likely among infants who co-sleep with their parents when the parents use recreational drugs or alcohol. Taking recreational drugs is clearly a bad idea for any parent, and now is the best time to kick the habit if you have not already done so.

STARTING OVER: RELACTATING AND RESUMING BREASTFEEDING

Mothers stop breastfeeding for a variety of reasons. Some may have decided against breastfeeding initially or experienced breastfeeding problems that led to unplanned early weaning. A separation from a baby due to hospitalization or other causes may have led to a decreasing milk supply despite pumping. An unaddressed imbalance in the breastfeeding rhythm or stress may have affected your milk let-down. Whatever the reason, it is sometimes possible to begin again, or *relactate*—if not always to completely nourish your child, at least enough to maintain the breastfeeding relationship. This may be especially important if you stopped breastfeeding only to find that your baby did not tolerate infant formulas.

Relactation works best if you either gave birth fairly recently (particularly if your child is less than three months old) or if your milk supply has been low or nonexistent for only a short period of time. While doctors may prescribe such drugs as metoclopramide to adoptive mothers who have not previously breastfed (see box on page 105) or to women attempting to relactate, the baby's frequent suckling and other forms of nipple stimulation, such as an electric breast pump, are critical to establishing or reestablishing milk supply.

If you are attempting to relactate, nurse your baby frequently, whenever he shows such hunger cues as a pursed mouth, sucking motions, or increased activity or alertness. You may need to nurse eight to ten or even more times per day, with two or more night feedings, for about fifteen to twenty minutes per session. If your baby is not eager to nurse as you are building your milk supply, provide him with positive reinforcement by using a nursing supplementer to provide formula or expressed or donor human milk. You should also stimulate your breasts with breast massage and a good-quality breast pump.

Don't expect this process to lead to instant results. Your baby may resist nursing for a week to two before he settles back down to breastfeeding, and it may take weeks for your milk supply to increase. To improve your chances of relactating, try to keep your nursing sessions relaxed and pleasurable for both you and your child. Drink enough fluids, and try to maintain an adequate diet. This is a process that will be much easier with the assistance of a lactation consultant. In addition, you might ask for help from your obstetrician or pediatric care provider, La Leche League volunteer, or family members and friends who may have experienced a similar situation.

Relactation does not always mean a return to exclusive breast-feeding. Since your milk production may well be lower than it was originally, you may need to supplement your baby's nutritional intake with formula, with breast milk from a donor milk bank, or with solid foods if he is older than six months. Meanwhile, it is crucial to monitor his weight gain and other signs that he is getting adequate calories and nutrition. Be sure that your pediatrician or family physician is aware of your breastfeeding situation and bring your child in for checkups as requested.

∞   GETTING HELP AND INFORMATION

No matter what your concerns may be about breastfeeding—whether your baby was born prematurely, you are worried about the effects of past breast surgery, or you wonder whether a disease or infection may be passed to your child through your breast milk—it is vital to communicate your complete medical history to your doctor and your child's pediatrician, making sure to emphasize your desire to breastfeed if at all possible. Since some medical professionals may not be as knowledgeable about the potential benefits of breastfeeding ill or very premature infants, you may need to provide them with information supporting your position. (Relevant information is available on the AAP website for parents, www.HealthyChildren.org, or from the La Leche League. See Appendix 1 for contact information.) If direct breastfeeding does not appear to be a possibility now or in the future, ask your pediatrician to help you explore the best alternatives—including expressing your breast milk for tube- or bottle-feeding; combining breast milk with additional formula-feeding; or feeding your infant breast milk obtained from a donor milk bank. The hospital where you give birth should provide you with a hospital-grade electric breast pump if you require one while you're there, but you will need a pump of your own once you're home. The hospital lactation specialist can help you locate one.

Inducing Lactation in Adoptive Mothers

A growing number of adoptive mothers are interested in breastfeeding their babies through induced lactation.

No drugs specifically designed to induce or enhance lactation have yet been approved by the FDA. However, a few medications typically prescribed for other reasons, such as the drug metoclopramide, have also been shown to stimulate or enhance milk production in some women. Such medications must be prescribed by a physician and do have side effects, so your doctor will want to review your medical history before prescribing them. In the United States and other countries, mothers have used herbal medications, available either in capsules or in teas, to stimulate or increase milk supply. Ask your doctor or lactation specialist about herbal medications before considering their use. (Note: herbal medications are not regulated in the United States for content, purity, or possible contaminants.)

You must accompany any medication with regular nipple and breast stimulation with a breast pump every two to three hours. Once your baby has arrived, he can be encouraged to suckle at the breast, initiating a breastfeeding relationship while further stimulating milk production. While there is no way to predict whether your milk production will reach sufficient levels to fully satisfy your baby's needs, many adoptive mothers happily breastfeed with the aid of a nursing supplementer that provides donor breast milk or formula.

If you're interested, you should talk to your doctor and start the process well before the arrival of the baby. Milk production can take weeks to begin—an average of four weeks—after you start pumping. The stress of the adoption process can also disrupt the production of milk.

THE REWARDS OF PERSISTENCE

Breastfeeding doesn't happen as naturally or easily for some women as others. An unexpected turn of events, a premature delivery, or illness in either the mother or the baby can temporarily change your plans to breastfeed. The good news is, most circumstances are a short-term setback. With some persistence—as well as the knowledge you've accumulated before you delivered—you'll soon realize that breastfeeding is possible even in situations that may seem overwhelming at first. That possibility can fuel your confidence that you will ultimately provide your baby with all the nutritional and health benefits of your breast milk. And you'll take pride in knowing that you did your best for your child.

CHAPTER 6

Going Home

After several days in the hospital, you're finally headed home, ready to begin life with your new addition. Gone will be the nurses, doctors, and health professionals who surrounded you during these first days with your baby. You'll be breastfeeding your baby on your own.

A HEALTHY START

Whether or not you have other children waiting for you, your return home will be a momentous occasion for you, your partner, and certainly your baby. You will begin or continue your family life together, and all the plans and expectations you have created for this time will—hopefully—start to fall into place. If this is your first child, you will need time to learn how to integrate breastfeeding into your everyday life. You will want to familiarize yourself with your baby's unique nursing style, respond to her changing feeding rhythms and needs, and learn how to meet your own needs for sleep, proper nutrition, and adult companionship in the process. If you have other children at home, you will need to do this while caring for the rest of your family. No matter what your home situation, you will want to allow time to adjust to your new circumstances, regain your strength and energy, practice the nursing techniques and positions you've recently learned, and get to know your new baby. This may sound overwhelming, but you will

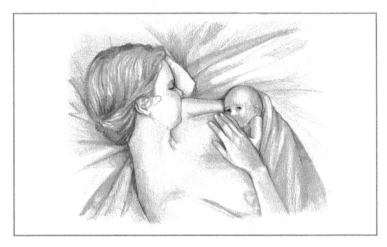

You and your partner can choose to make breastfeeding a time when you are all together and receive encouragement and support.

learn how to handle it. For most women the pleasures of breastfeeding—knowing they are giving their babies the best possible introduction to life, feeling the closeness to their newborns that nursing brings, and experiencing motherhood in this most natural of ways—make the effort more than worthwhile. Take advantage of this precious time with your newborn baby.

A SPECIAL PLACE FOR A SPECIAL TIME: ESTABLISHING A NURSING ROUTINE

It is such a joy to observe an infant's responses to the world. As you watch your newborn gaze in wonder at the people and objects around him, nestle against you with a whimper of pleasure, and occasionally startle in response to a loud noise, you may feel that you're experiencing many of the wide range of emotions yourself. During the first days and weeks at home with a new baby, you may swing between feelings of joy and uncertainty, confidence and confusion, excitement and exasperation. These are all very natural and expected feelings. If your emotional responses during the postpartum period are more extreme than you expected or feel you can handle, you should notify your physician. In general, the simpler and more predictable you can keep your daily routine as you continue getting to know your baby and familiarizing yourself with breastfeeding, the better for you and your family.

You Feed the Baby with Your Body?

MANAGING OLDER SIBLINGS

Many women who breastfeed their newborns wonder how their older children will respond to nursing sessions and worry about how to keep older siblings occupied during frequent early breastfeeding sessions. It's safe to assume that all your children will show a healthy curiosity about this amazing and beautiful manner of feeding a brand-new baby. As long as you explain the nursing process in simple language and maintain a matter-of-fact approach to their questions and their desire to watch the baby breastfeed, such "family time" may turn out to be a positive and educational experience for all.

Don't be surprised if your older children tend to hover nearby during nursing sessions or even try to climb into your lap. Include them if you can by talking about how you used to breastfeed them (if you did), giving them a little hug with your free arm, telling them a story, or watching while they draw you a picture, work in a workbook, or play with a toy. You might also read one of the children's books about breastfeeding listed in Appendix 1. Some mothers find that nursing sessions are wonderful times to listen to music or children's stories with their babies' siblings. In this way, nursing time can be used to draw closer to all the children, not just the new one. Older children may also be grateful for the chance to express the feelings of closeness that breastfeeding inspires by folding laundry nearby, getting you a glass of water, holding the baby while you prepare to nurse, or otherwise contributing to their family's care.

If your toddler or preschooler asks if she can try nursing, the choice is obviously yours. In most cases, a child who is no longer breastfed may find the experience too strange to try more than once. She will probably not remember how to nurse and will run off, satisfied, after a quick experiment.

If you already have a nursing toddler who may not want to relinquish the breast when your new baby enters the family, or if you feel that this is not the time to begin weaning, you may decide to *tandem-nurse*—breastfeed both the toddler and the newborn. If so, be sure to inform your newborn's pediatrician of your decision so your infant's growth can be monitored more closely. Keep in mind that while the older child can receive foods and liquids from other sources, your infant depends entirely on your breast milk for her nutrition. Therefore, you should offer the breast to your infant first, and nurse your older child only after your infant has had her fill. Also watch your own nutrition and energy levels more closely. You will need to eat well enough to support the production of extra breast milk and get the additional rest necessary to handle the extra demands on your body. Your baby's pediatrician will be aware of all of these issues and can help you deal with them. You may wonder whether the newborn will still receive the advantages of colostrum during tandem nursing. Analysis of mother's milk shows that a mother who delivers a newborn does produce colostrum and milk designed to meet the needs of the newborn, even though the mother is still nursing a toddler. This offers the desired advantages for the newborn but no adverse consequences for the older child.

Though one of the great advantages of breastfeeding is its adaptability—you can feed your baby practically anywhere without equipment and without delay—you might find that choosing one or two favorite places for breastfeeding at first will make your adjustment easier. During the day, you might opt for a sofa or chair in the living room or kitchen, since this allows you to take part in family life as you nurse. Some new mothers find that breastfeeding in bed, with plenty of pillows for support and their baby's bassinet waiting close by, allows the baby to drift off comfortably to sleep at the end of the nursing session and makes it easier for the mother to nap.

Nursing mothers in many cultures sleep with their babies until they wean. The American Academy of Pediatrics, however, has expressed concern that bed sharing is hazardous. Bed sharing is a particular concern if the mother is obese; if she is using any substances that may alter her state of arousal, such as mind-altering drugs or excessive alcohol; if she is a smoker; or if other children are also in

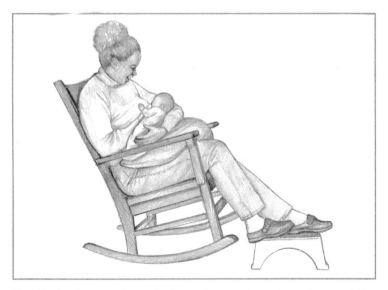

Transitioning from nursing at the hospital to nursing at home is an enriching and rewarding experience.

the bed. If you decide to let your infant sleep in your bed, *never* place him in a facedown position. Always place him on his back. Avoid soft surfaces, loose pillows, or loose covers, and move the bed away from the wall and other furniture to keep your baby from becoming trapped. Never put your baby to sleep on a waterbed. Consider moving him to his bassinet, on his back, after breastfeeding and before you drift off to sleep. It is also risky to fall asleep with your infant on a couch or in a reclining chair. The American Academy of Pediatrics recommends parents have their new babies sleep in the same room as the parents, but on a separate sleep surface, such as a bassinet.

Once you've picked a couple of locations for breastfeeding, make sure that such essentials as baby wipes and diapers are within reach before you start nursing. Keep a bottle of water or something else to drink nearby for you, as nursing mothers should drink plenty of water or other noncaffeinated beverages to avoid thirst. If you have older children, a basket of toys, workbooks, or audio recordings can keep you from having to get up in the middle of a breastfeeding session. You might also keep a pad and pencil within reach to track your baby's feedings (you can also use the breast-feeding record in Appendix 2). Finally, while studies have shown that eye contact and other communication during feedings benefit your infant's brain development (and is rewarding for you too), you may want to keep a book, magazine, or the television remote control within reach for those times when he falls asleep in your arms. Of course, you won't necessarily need every one of these items, nor do you need to create a formal "nursing area" to breast-feed successfully, but thinking ahead about what you might want nearby can make life more manageable in the early days.

ꭗ   FINDING TIME ALONE

Once you have started breastfeeding at home, you may feel as though you never stop—particularly during the first week or two. Though breastfed babies show a wide range of normal feeding pat-

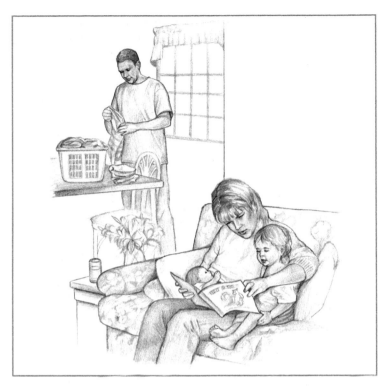

Some nursing sessions provide a great opportunity to spend time with the entire family.

terns (and these patterns frequently differ even day to day), many babies begin feeding every hour or two as they learn to suckle effectively and as your milk supply becomes established. While not all of these sessions will be full feedings (you may have a baby who enjoys "snacking" frequently), healthy newborns breastfeed about eight to twelve times per day—that is, once every two or three hours on average. In many cases, daytime feedings may be less than two hours apart, leaving time for somewhat longer periods of sleep at night. It is easy to see, then, why new mothers who breastfeed postpone plans to send out baby announcements, finish the nursery, or entertain visitors until about two to three weeks after birth.

By focusing on your relationship with your newborn, you can make sure that your milk supply is established, your breastfeeding relationship is securely in place, you baby is receiving the nutrition he needs, and the two of you are communicating well.

Home, but Not Alone

GETTING THE HELP YOU REALLY NEED

Everyone loves a newborn, and you may find yourself besieged with well-wishers once you have returned home with your baby. Support is always welcome, of course, but when it interferes with your developing breastfeeding relationship (when a relative offers to give the baby a bottle of formula, juice, or water, for example, so that you can "get some rest"), you will need to excuse yourself and your infant from the celebration or redirect your visitors' energy. Try asking helpers who want to feed the baby to prepare meals for the family instead, spend time with older children, do the laundry, or entertain other visitors while you and your baby take a nap. If your mother or mother-in-law longs to cuddle her new grandchild, ask her to hold the baby while you take a shower or get dressed. If you find you are having trouble with breastfeeding or other new parenting skills, a visitor who is an experienced breastfeeding mother may be able to help you enormously during this period. If you know that your helper's knowledge in this area is limited, however, or she does not agree with your philosophy regarding breastfeeding, quietly turn to your "official" support system (your child's pediatrician or family physician, your La Leche League volunteer, or a lactation specialist) instead. Of course, you can still appreciate and thank your friend for her efforts.

Often it's not easy to enjoy a private "honeymoon" with your newborn. The baby's father naturally wants to establish a relationship with his infant and to spend time with you. Friends and relatives are eager to see the baby and offer all kinds of parenting advice. Your other children not only will want to play with the baby but also may need and demand more attention as they watch you tending to their new sibling. Of course, such needs must be met to some degree. But just as you needed to look out for your newborn's needs in the hospital, it's important to limit your interactions, as well as your baby's, with others for the two or three weeks it takes to establish your daily rhythm. Restrict visitors to the one or two people who you think will really be able to help with household management (while leaving much of the baby cuddling to you), and schedule visits with others for a month from now or even later. Use voice mail to screen calls so that you can get enough sleep and save your energy for your baby. As far as sleep goes, consider napping yourself whenever your newborn sleeps. Resist the urge to try to get household chores done when your baby is sleeping. If you have hired a professional helper or baby nurse, make sure she focuses on freeing you up from household and social obligations, so that you have little to worry about besides caring for yourself and your infant, establishing a breastfeeding rhythm, eating well, and getting enough sleep. Ask your partner, relatives, or friends to help with the other children.

SETTLING IN: THE FIRST FEW WEEKS OF BREASTFEEDING

The first weeks of breastfeeding are a fascinating time of transition for you as well as your baby. During this time you will learn what it feels like to breastfeed, how to recognize your baby's hunger signals, and how to know when your let-down or milk ejection reflex has occurred (see Chapter 2). You will learn whether your baby is a frequent snacker or prefers less frequent but longer meals, whether nursing tends to put her to sleep or to stimulate her, and whether she enjoys pausing occasionally to exchange looks with you or focuses entirely upon nursing until she's had her fill. She will not always breastfeed in the same way, of course—just as you will not always be in the same mood each time you nurse. But you will begin to recognize and respond to breastfeeding cues. As you do so, the two of you will gradually grow more comfortable together, respond to each other's signals more effectively, and develop a unique breastfeeding rhythm.

Ideally, by the time you arrive home your baby will already have learned to latch on to the breast properly. (If she hasn't, it's very important to address this issue immediately by reviewing the instructions in Chapter 4 and asking for help from your baby's pediatrician, your La Leche League volunteer, or a lactation specialist.) Your newborn may even prefer one breast at this point, tending to nurse longer on one than on the other. It is a good idea to let her nurse as long as she wants. Keep in mind that once your mature milk comes in, its content changes during the course of a single breastfeeding from the somewhat watery *foremilk* to the creamier, fat-rich *hindmilk,* which, like any good dessert, leaves your baby feeling content and sleepy. By allowing your baby to nurse until she's satisfied (once she's latched on properly), you can ensure that she will receive all the benefits of breast milk.

Even if she clearly prefers one breast over the other, however, it's important to alternate the breast you offer first with each breastfeeding session. This ensures that a full milk supply is stimulated for both breasts and that as much milk as possible has been removed from each. At first, to remember which breast to start with, consider moving a safety pin from one side of your nursing bra to the other after each feeding. Later on you will know which breast feels fuller and start the next feeding there.

☙   IS SHE EATING WELL?

As you feed your baby, continue to look for signs of correct nursing. In addition to making sure she is latched on properly, with her mouth around as much of the areola as possible, you should hear her swallow as her mouth fills with milk. During the first few days she may not swallow as often, since the volume of the colostrum she is ingesting is still low. After the second to fifth day following childbirth, however, your milk will have increased in volume and your baby should be swallowing after every one or two sucks once the milk has let down. While she is nursing, you may see some milk escaping from around her lips or notice that milk is dripping from your other breast. These are good signs that your let-down reflex is working properly (see below) and your body is producing the breast milk your baby needs. After a nursing session, your infant should appear content and satisfied. If she continues to fuss, she may want to return to the breast for more milk, need to burp, need her diaper changed, or simply want to be held and cuddled.

It is important during this early period to breastfeed your baby whenever she shows signs of hunger, rather than delaying in an effort to stick to a set schedule. Don't wait for her to cry for a feeding; bring her to the breast as soon as you see increased activity or alertness. Keep in mind that the more frequently your baby nurses, the more she will stimulate your milk production and the more easily and quickly the two of you will reach a satisfactory balance of milk supply and demand. If your baby tends to sleep for long periods or is simply undemanding, you may need to encourage her to feed more often than she would naturally. Wake her up for a feeding after four hours of sleep, initiate breastfeeding every few hours whether or not she acts hungry on her own, and continue nursing for at least ten minutes (and preferably longer) to ensure that she gets plenty of milk. It is also best to avoid pacifiers for at least the first month or so to encourage your baby to do all her suckling at the breast.

CHECKING HER DIAPER

Some of the best signs that your baby is breastfeeding successfully can be found in her diaper. As your milk supply becomes more abundant, your breastfeeding baby will wet more diapers per day. By five to seven days after birth, she should be wetting her diaper at least six to eight times in a twenty-four-hour period. You may have to look closely to tell whether a highly absorbent disposable diaper is wet. Comparing the weight of a fresh diaper to the one you are removing can help you decide if the baby has urinated in it. Coinciding with the increase in your milk volume (generally after the second to fifth day), you should also notice that the urine is colorless or pale yellow—not dark yellow or red- or pink-speckled. (The latter are signs of highly concentrated urine, which may be normal in the first few days after delivery but later could mean that your baby is not getting enough milk.) Once your milk volume increases, your infant should also pass about three or four bowel movements each day. These stools will consist of loose yellow curds—no longer the tarry black stool of the first few days—and much of the normal watery stool may be absorbed into a diaper, leaving what appears to be a stain. Some infants pass a yellow stool after each feeding at this point, and this is considered perfectly normal during the early weeks. After about a month the number of bowel movements will start to decrease. Babies older than one month will sometimes go for days or even a week or more without passing a stool. This, too, is normal, as long as she still feeds eagerly, is gaining weight well, has a soft tummy, and has a soft, usually large stool when she does have one. Anytime you have concerns about your baby's stool or urination patterns, consult your pediatric health care provider.

∞   WEIGHT GAIN

While diapers can provide important clues that a baby is not getting enough to eat, your baby's weight gain remains the most reliable sign of breastfeeding success. A breastfeeding baby who is getting enough milk will gain weight, while a baby who is not nursing well will not gain as well or may even lose weight. Most babies lose up to 7 percent of their birth weight in the first few days after birth (with larger babies tending to lose more weight than smaller ones), but this weight loss should stop once your milk production increases, beginning around the second to fifth day following childbirth. At that time, your infant should start regaining her lost weight right away. She will usually exceed her birth weight between ten to fourteen days after birth. From about her fifth day of life through her third month, she should gain ½ ounce to 1 ounce per day, or ½ to 1 pound every two weeks. Your pediatrician will weigh your baby during the initial newborn checkup, a couple of days after you return home from the hospital.

∞ YOUR BREASTS

Your breasts can also provide a great deal of information about how well your breastfeeding relationship with your baby is progressing. As we pointed out in Chapter 2, your breasts should increase in size and feel heavier about two to five days after delivery—a signal that your milk is transitioning in composition and increasing in volume. At feeding times, your breasts may become so full and firm that your baby has trouble latching on correctly. In this case, you may need to hand-express or pump a little milk for a few minutes to soften them (see Chapter 9). If you have any trouble managing this or your baby still cannot latch on, ask your pediatrician, a lactation specialist, or an experienced friend for help right away. It is important for your baby to continue to breastfeed as frequently as she wants to during this period, when your level of milk production is being established.

Once your baby latches on properly and begins to nurse, you may feel the tingly pins-and-needles sensation of the milk let-down or milk ejection reflex. This reflex—a physiological response to your baby's stimulation of your nipples while feeding—causes your milk to flow more plentifully, providing your baby with the abundant milk she needs. The milk ejection reflex should be noticeable to most mothers by about two weeks after delivery. In the early days after childbirth, when oxytocin is released in your body in response to your baby's feeding, you may also notice cramping in your lower abdomen. In fact, some women primarily note the uterine contractions, as opposed to the squeezing sensation in their breasts, in the early days after delivery. The cramping is a good sign, even though it may produce temporary discomfort. These contractions of the muscles of your uterus help it return to its pre-pregnancy size, preventing excessive uterine bleeding.

Once your baby has nursed fully on each breast, your breasts will feel soft again—letting you know that your baby has had an adequate feeding. By about two to three weeks after birth, your breasts will feel not quite as excessively firm between feedings, but a milder fluctuation between fullness before feeding and softening after feeding will continue throughout your months or years of nursing. Anytime you miss a feeding or have a longer delay than usual between feedings, you will experience a notable fullness in your lactating breasts. As your breastfeeding relationship develops, you will look forward to nursing sessions as a way to ease your breasts' fullness as well as a way to nurture and spend time with your baby.

⌒⌒ NIPPLE TENDERNESS

Many mothers worry that nipple tenderness automatically means something is wrong with the way their babies are nursing. While extremely painful nipples indicate that your baby is not latching on correctly or that some other problem needs attention (such as an infection—see Chapter 8), a certain amount of nipple sensitivity or tenderness is common during the early days of breastfeeding. This is true even among mothers who are nursing successfully, especially if they live in an area with a dry climate. Usually this sensitivity fades after the first few suckles on the breast and disappears completely after the first week or so. If you find that your nipples have become raw, are cracked, or are bleeding, try soothing them with colostrum or human milk, which can be expressed and spread over the nipples. An alternative treatment is to apply purified, medical-grade lanolin (available at your local pharmacy) after you feed the baby. Allow the nipple to air-dry first. Exposing the nipples to air instead of keeping them covered constantly may also help to keep your nipples healthy. Refer to Chapter 8 for more pointers and ask your pediatrician for advice. Keep in mind that preventing or treating nipple soreness involves working with your baby to make sure that he is latching on by taking as much of the areola into his wide-open mouth as possible and is not just sucking on the nipple. Rotating the positions you use when feeding your baby will also help.

∞   THE FIRST CHECKUP

While all of these signs and conditions are useful ways to monitor your baby's and your own breastfeeding progress, there is no substitute for that first visit to your child's pediatrician, no later than two or three days after your discharge from the hospital. By having your baby weighed, your breasts assessed, your breastfeeding observed, and your questions answered at this early stage, most potential breastfeeding problems can be prevented or corrected before they cause any lasting damage.

During your early visits to the pediatrician, you should check with your doctor about vitamin D supplements for your baby. Vitamin D is typically made by exposing the skin to sunlight. Due to concerns about sun exposure increasing risk of skin cancer over time, the American Academy of Pediatrics recommends a vitamin D supplement, beginning within days after birth for the exclusively breastfed infant, instead of exposing the baby's skin to natural sunlight. Additionally, all children receiving less than 32 ounces of vitamin-D-fortified formula (for infants less than one year of age) or 32 ounces of vitamin-D-fortified cow's milk (for the child older than one year) daily should receive a supplement of vitamin D. Your pediatrician is your best source for discussing all aspects of infant nutrition.

When to Call an Expert

WARNING SIGNS OF PROBLEMS IN BREASTFEEDING

Natural as the breastfeeding process is, problems can occasionally arise. When they do surface, they may grow worse very quickly and interfere with your milk production or your baby's ability to get the nutrition she needs. For this reason, it's vital to get help right away if you experience difficulty with breastfeeding at home or observe any of the symptoms listed below. Contact your baby's pediatrician, and don't stop asking for one-on-one guidance until you get the help you need.

- **Your baby's nursing sessions are either very short or extremely long.** Breastfeeding sessions that are consistently briefer than about ten minutes during the first few months may mean that your baby isn't getting enough milk and that not enough milk is being removed to stimulate your ongoing milk production. Sessions that last consistently longer than about fifty minutes may mean that your baby isn't receiving enough milk due to ineffective suckling or low milk production.
- **Your baby still seems hungry after most feedings.** She may not be ingesting enough milk. Consult your pediatrician and have her weighed right away. Meanwhile, double-check her latch-on and position at the breast to try to increase the milk she is getting.
- **Your newborn frequently misses nursing sessions or sleeps through the night.** Frequent feedings around the clock are a necessary part of breastfeeding a new baby. Your baby requires a feeding every few hours to gain sufficient weight to thrive. If your newborn sleeps longer than four hours a night, wake her up and encourage her to nurse.

- You don't hear frequent swallowing when your baby nurses after your milk supply has come in. Your baby will probably swallow occasionally as she begins to nurse, more frequently as she continues a session, and less frequently again near the end. Swallowing is an excellent sign that she is actually ingesting milk, and its absence should prompt you to call her pediatrician at once. (Remember, though, that you may not be able to hear your baby swallowing when she is taking small sips of colostrum in the early days.)

- By two weeks of age, your baby is under her birth weight or hasn't started gaining at least 5 to 7 ounces per week since your milk came in. Inadequate weight gain is one of the strongest indicators that a baby is not getting enough milk.

- After seven days, your baby has fewer than six wet diapers and four stools per day, her urine is dark yellow or specked with red, or her stools are still dark rather than yellow and loose. If you or your pediatrician is concerned about your child's milk intake, you might want to keep a written record of your baby's wet diapers and bowel movements during the early days to be sure she is progressing properly. Most hospitals and lactation specialists can provide you with a special diary to use in recording your newborn's feedings and diaper changes, or you can use the one in Appendix 2.

- After five days, your milk hasn't come in or your breasts don't feel as though they're filling with milk. If you feel this way, have your baby weighed by her pediatrician immediately. This is the most precise way to tell whether she is ingesting enough milk. You may also want to have your breasts examined.

- You experience severe breast engorgement. Hard, painful breasts may prevent your baby from latching on correctly and discourage both of you from nursing. You may need to express milk manually or with an electric breast pump until your breasts have softened somewhat. Severe, unrelieved engorgement can decrease your milk supply.

- **The fullness and hardness of your breasts don't decrease by the end of a feeding.** Your baby may not be drinking enough milk or may be suckling ineffectively.
- **Severe pain interferes with breastfeeding.** Your baby is probably not latching on correctly. If you have severe nipple pain or significant cracking of the nipples that makes it too painful to nurse, consult your physician or lactation specialist. She can check for a nipple or breast infection such as mastitis (see Chapter 8) and help you with any problems with latching on. You may need to start breastfeeding on the less sore side or even use an electric breast pump until your nipples have healed. Your lactation specialist or La Leche volunteer can show you how to do this.
- **After a week or two, you don't notice the sensations associated with your milk let-down reflex.** Though this may not indicate a problem at all, it could mean that your milk production is low. Ask your baby's pediatrician to evaluate her and observe your breastfeeding technique. Your local La Leche League volunteer or lactation specialist can help assess the situation, too.

FINDING YOUR RHYTHM: ENJOYING LIFE AS A BREASTFEEDING MOTHER

As with most things we do, there is no substitute for time and experience in perfecting your breastfeeding technique. Focusing on your baby for the first weeks at home will add to your confidence and your infant's ability to master the basics of his new environment. By the second or third month, you will have become familiar with your baby's breastfeeding "personality"—whether he is an eager, lip-smacking nurser or a drowsy, dreamy type who needs to be wakened occasionally to finish a feeding. You will recognize his typical early signs of hunger (lip and tongue movements, rooting, waving fists, alert and eager looking around) and put him to the breast before he begins his cry of hunger. His feedings will decrease in frequency but perhaps increase in length as he takes advantage of long, leisurely sessions that give him all the nutrients he needs. While no set number of breastfeeding sessions is "right" for every nursing baby, you will soon grow accustomed to the number that is right for your child. Throughout the months ahead, his demand for food will surge and decline as he experiences growth spurts or varying levels of physical activity. Growth spurts typically occur around three weeks, six weeks, three months, and six months of age, although this varies from baby to baby. During a growth spurt your baby may seem to want to nurse almost continuously. Typically this will last only for about two or three days. Then he will be back to his own routine and so will you. It is very important to understand that if you give extra formula during this time instead of breastfeeding more, the baby will not help your body make more breast milk to keep up with his growing needs. Your early observation and experience of his typical behavior (along with the information provided in Chapter 9 and the advice of your pediatrician) will help you understand when these changes are natural aspects of your child's development and when they require treatment or some other response.

⊙ REJOINING THE OUTSIDE WORLD

When you and your baby have settled into a comfortable routine, you may feel the urge to rejoin the outside world—to introduce your baby to those you love and to interact with other adults yourself. This transition should not be difficult as long as you are getting the sleep and nutrition you need to sustain your milk production and keep your energy level up.

Am I Spoiling Him?

BREASTFEEDING ON DEMAND

As relatives and friends observe your readiness to respond to your child's frequent demands for feedings, you may hear a comment or two about "spoiling" your child. This response to breastfeeding on demand results from widespread confusion between meeting a baby's genuine needs and allowing an older child to indulge in self-defeating behavior. By feeding your baby whenever he shows hunger (even if that's every one or two hours), you are teaching him that his needs will be met and that his parents are listening to him. Responding to a baby's cues will result not in a spoiled child but rather in a confident and trusting one. And since breast milk is easier to digest than formula, it's normal for breastfed babies to want to eat more frequently than formula-fed babies.

Breastfeeding a baby while resuming your pre-baby life should become routine relatively quickly once you are comfortable with several breastfeeding positions and different nursing clothes. You will discover some great advantages of breastfeeding—how easy it is to pick up and go when there are no bottles to prepare and no pacifiers to search for. And life is much less expensive when you don't have to stock up on formula every week. Getting out and about with a breastfed baby is easier now that breastfeeding in public is becoming a common and accepted practice virtually everywhere across the country, thanks in part to a surge of state and federal legislation protecting mothers' rights to breastfeed wherever they like.

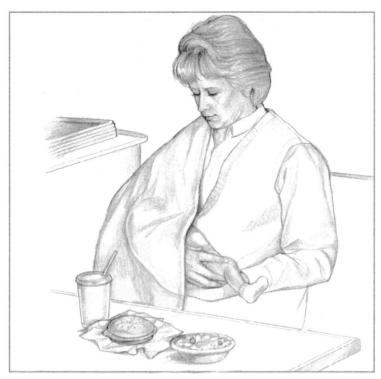

A blanket or sling can help you nurse discreetly in public.

Still, you may encounter the occasional challenge to your new lifestyle. Critics may admonish you for nursing in public, ask you when you plan to wean your baby (even when he's just months old), or suggest you offer the baby a bottle of formula if your milk doesn't let down readily when your baby wants to nurse. (Even after several months, glitches occur occasionally in your supply-and-demand relationship with your baby as he experiences a growth spurt, you go through a stressful period, or other life events occur.) You may find situations where you just don't feel at all comfortable breastfeeding while others are present, especially in the early weeks as you and your baby are learning your new breast-feeding skills. In these cases, simply excuse yourself and go to another area to nurse, or express your breast milk ahead of time and feed it to your baby in a bottle when you need to after the baby is three to four weeks old. (See Chapter 9 for tips on expressing and storing human milk.)

Around this time, you may wonder how you will adjust to working while continuing to breastfeed. (Reading Chapter 10 ahead of time can start you on the road to meeting this challenge.) You may be separated from your baby for longer periods, requiring you to provide one or more bottles of expressed breast milk to your infant's caregiver in your absence. Planning ahead, along with the solid base of breastfeeding experience you've acquired, will help you adjust to whatever changes occur. Once you have committed yourself to nurturing your baby in the best way you can, little can stand in the way of a lasting and fulfilling breastfeeding relationship.

∞   WHAT ABOUT BIRTH CONTROL?

Once you have settled into life as a breastfeeding mother, you will no doubt enjoy renewing your relationship with your partner as well. One of the welcome advantages of exclusive round-the-clock breastfeeding (no water, juice, formula, solids, or other supplements for the baby) is that it significantly reduces the chance of your becoming pregnant again during the first six months because it delays the resumption of your ovulatory cycles. If your baby is less than six months old, your periods have not yet started again, *and* you are fully breastfeeding both day and night, you will *probably* not become pregnant even without the active use of contraceptive methods.

At about six weeks postpartum, once your milk supply is firmly established, you may begin using contraceptives, but be sure to discuss the issue with your infant's pediatrician and your gynecologist first. As we pointed out in Chapter 5, there are no harmful effects on infants when the mother uses hormonal contraceptives, but their use may diminish milk supply, especially during the early weeks of breastfeeding. This is especially true when hormonal contraception is combined with stressors such as a return to work or less-frequent breastfeeding. Birth control pills with high doses of estrogen are more likely to decrease milk supply. Condoms, a diaphragm, or a cervical cap and spermicide may be considered as alternative choices for now (even if somewhat less effective), since these forms of birth control are unlikely to interfere with your milk supply.

Q & A

Can I Handle This?

Q: *I lose track of how often my baby has breastfed on a given day or how many wet diapers she's had. Also, I have a hard time telling the difference between a "snack" and a real feeding. Is it important to pay attention to this?*

A: Since breastfeeding involves no bottles with milk measured in visible ounces, it is important to monitor your baby's milk intake in other ways —particularly during the early weeks and months of life. The best way to make sure your baby is eating enough is to have her weight checked regularly—at every visit to the pediatrician and even between visits if your pediatrician recommends it. In the meantime, try keeping a breastfeeding log or diary to note each nursing session and wet diaper. There's no need to be obsessive about this, but spot-checking can be very reassuring as you establish your milk supply, and the information is useful to share with your pediatrician.

Q: *My mother-in-law did not nurse her children and feels very uncomfortable with my nursing. She's supportive in her way but wants to feed my two-week-old a bottle. Should I give in and let her do this?*

A: It's more important to establish and maintain your breastfeeding relationship with your infant right now than it is for your mother-in-law to feed her. Try suggesting other ways to bond with her grandchild, such as cuddling her between nursing sessions, taking her for a stroll, bathing her, or changing her diaper. Explain to her how important it is for you to breastfeed exclusively, point out the many advantages breastfeeding provides for your baby, and ask her to help you by respecting your wishes.

Q: *My baby is four weeks old, and already I feel like I'm suffering from extreme sleep deprivation. How can I breastfeed on demand and still get enough sleep?*

A: You can minimize sleep disruption by keeping your baby close by the bed in her own bassinet. (See pages 111–112 for the AAP's recommendations regarding safe sleep habits for mother and baby.) With your baby beside you, you need only roll over, pick her up, and place her next to you to breastfeed. If your partner is willing to change the baby's diaper when necessary, you can fall back asleep once a nursing session is over. Also, try to develop the habit of sleeping during the day when the baby sleeps. Some sleep deprivation is always part of the process of early parenting, but breastfeeding certainly disrupts sleep less than getting up and preparing a bottle of formula. And soon your baby will sleep for longer intervals.

A HEALTHY FAMILY: BREASTFEEDING FOR LIFE

Making the decision to breastfeed your baby is a major commitment and one that has important ramifications for you, your baby, and your family. Remember that the first few weeks are about helping your baby learn to nurse and learning how best to respond to this new person. Once you know each other better, nursing becomes simple.

It helps to have the support of your family, especially your partner. Now that you're in the throes of nursing an infant, you are probably experiencing the rewards of that support, which hopefully will go beyond your family to include your friends, your employer, and others you see regularly. With their support, your newfound confidence, and the special relationship you've forged with your infant, your baby is on his way to a healthy start.

CHAPTER 7

Good Nutrition Helps

You're on your way out the door when you realize you forgot to eat breakfast. You grab a muffin, down some juice, and then head out for the day with your baby in tow. You figure the multivitamin you take every day will give you the nutrients you need. Not so. When it comes to healthy eating—both for you and your baby—there is simply no replacement for proper nourishment with good food.

YOU ARE WHAT YOU EAT

Your own first months with your newborn have no doubt been an exhilarating experience for you both, but this period can also be tiring and even stressful. With round-the-clock infant care as your top priority and other aspects of life clamoring for attention, it's not always easy to pay attention to your own needs. Fortunately, your body has been preparing for breastfeeding since before childbirth without requiring any special diet or additional nutritional help other than a daily prenatal vitamin or a multivitamin/mineral supplement. You will both get all the nutrients you need as long as you eat a healthy diet that includes a good variety of foods in more or less the correct amounts. This basic diet will provide you with all the calcium, iron, protein, and other vital nutrients to meet your needs.

To many new mothers—particularly those who are eager to return to somewhere near their pre-pregnancy weight—the volume of food recommended looks like a lot. Keep in mind, though, that

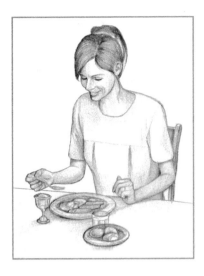

Eating a balanced diet provides your body with the nutrients it needs for breastfeeding and good health.

Dietary Guidelines for Americans

KEY RECOMMENDATIONS

- Increase consumption of vegetables and fruits, selecting a wide variety.
- Increase consumption of whole-grain products and total dietary fiber.
- Increase consumption of reduced-fat milk and dairy products.
- Consume moderate amounts of lean meat, poultry, and eggs. Incorporate more fish into the diet.
- Get adequate amounts of vitamin D, calcium, and potassium.
- Limit saturated fats, trans fats, cholesterol, salt (sodium), alcohol, and added sugars.

Source: U.S. Department of Agriculture (www.dietaryguidelines.gov)

a serving as described here is not a plateful. One serving of breads and grains, for example, is 1 slice of bread, ½ bagel, or ½ cup of cooked rice. Since each group contains a wide variety of delicious foods, you should be able to find a number of dishes you enjoy. In the bread and grain group, for example, you can satisfy your daily requirement with hot cereal (½ cup per serving), pasta (½ cup per serving), whole-grain crackers (4 per serving), or even a corn tortilla (1 per serving).

HOW A HEALTHY DIET HELPS YOU BREASTFEED

For centuries, new mothers have been promised that certain foods or regimens will increase their milk production, stimulate their babies' development, or speed their own return to their prepregnancy state. We now know that a normal, healthy diet is all it really takes for a breastfeeding mother to maintain her milk supply and sustain both her baby's and her own health. Still, certain components of this normal diet are especially important when your body is producing milk.

☞   CALCIUM

Calcium is among the most important minerals in your diet. Your body stores of calcium (primarily from your bones) supply much of the calcium in your breast milk to meet your baby's calcium needs. Studies show that women lose 3 to 5 percent of their bone mass when they are breastfeeding. After you finish breastfeeding, your body must replenish the calcium that was used to produce your milk. Making sure you consume the recommended amount of calcium in a normal diet—1,000 milligrams daily for all women ages eighteen to fifty and 1,300 milligrams for teenage mothers—helps ensure that your bones will remain strong after you have weaned your baby. The good news is that you recover the bone lost during breastfeeding within the six-month period after you wean your baby.

By consuming three servings of dairy products—8 ounces of

Don't Forget Water!

YOUR LIQUID INTAKE

Contrary to popular belief, no particular food or ingredient is guaranteed to increase your milk supply—but an inadequate supply of liquids can negatively affect your milk production and leave you feeling depleted. Whether you prefer water, milk, juice, or non-caffeinated sodas, keep something to drink nearby while you breastfeed, and make a habit of drinking enough to prevent becoming thirsty. All healthy adults are encouraged to drink between 6 and 8 glasses of fluids per day. It is not recommended that you force fluids beyond your usual thirst. You should remember, however, that by the time you feel thirsty, you are likely to be mildly dehydrated. If your urine is dark yellow or you are constipated, you may not be getting enough fluid.

milk is one serving—per day, you should receive the calcium you need. If you dislike milk, you can get the calcium you need from cheese and yogurt. If you are allergic to dairy products, try calcium-fortified juice, tofu, dark leafy greens such as spinach and kale, broccoli, or dried beans. You can also get calcium in fortified foods such as breakfast cereal. (Contrary to popular myth, it is not necessary to drink milk to make milk.) If you do not routinely consume 1,000 milligrams of calcium in your diet, talk to your doctor or nutritionist about a dietary supplement of calcium. (Avoid supplements made from crushed oyster shells, though, because of concern about lead from these sources.) Consuming 1,000 milligrams of calcium daily—not only while breastfeeding but throughout life until you reach menopause—will decrease your risk of osteoporosis in later life.

∞   VITAMIN D

Vitamin D—often known as the "sunshine vitamin"—is just as important as calcium when it comes to maintaining bone strength. Vitamin D is essential for absorbing dietary calcium from your intestinal tract. The amount of vitamin D you need depends on whom you ask. Most experts currently recommend getting at least 400 IU of vitamin D a day, but some suggest getting as much as 1,000 IU. Exposure to sunlight is one of the best ways to get your vitamin D, but it's not the safest, given concerns about skin cancer. It's also unreliable and depends a great deal on where you live. Instead, you should look to get vitamin D from foods such as salmon, mackerel, fortified milk or orange juice, and yogurt. Some ready-to-eat breakfast cereals are fortified with vitamin D. You can get vitamin D from supplements, too.

Keep in mind, though, that your baby still needs vitamin D supplementation, even if you're taking a supplement. Breast milk does not provide babies with enough vitamin D. Exclusively breastfed infants or those getting less than 32 ounces of vitamin-D-fortified formula per day need 400 IU of vitamin D per day, because sunlight exposure can no longer be safely recommended as their primary source of vitamin D. Babies exclusively breastfed may develop a condition called rickets when adequate vitamin D is not provided. Make sure to talk to your baby's doctor about the need for supplementation.

∞   PROTEIN

Protein is another component of a healthy diet that demands your attention while you are breastfeeding. Protein builds, repairs, and maintains body tissues. You need 6 to 6 ½ ounces a day when you're nursing. You can get it best by eating two or three servings of lean meat, poultry, or fish, usually about 3 ounces (the size of a deck of cards) in a serving. You can also get 1-ounce equivalents of protein from 1 egg, 1 tablespoon of peanut butter, nuts (12 almonds or 24 pistachios, for instance), or dried beans (¼ cup cooked). It's also a good idea to include fish in your weekly diet as one source of protein, especially fatty fish such as salmon, tuna, and mackerel. These types of fish are rich sources of DHA (docosahexaenoic acid), an omega-3 fatty acid that is found in breast milk and contributes to growth and development of an infant's brain and eyes. In addition, DHA content of milk declines with breastfeeding and can be replenished by eating fatty fish. As always, it's best to vary your choices as much as possible, while keeping saturated fat intake to moderate levels. To do that, choose lean meats or low-fat varieties whenever possible.

Since peanuts are one of the foods most likely to cause an allergic response in both children and adults, be sure to monitor your baby's response when you eat foods containing peanuts, especially if there is a family history of food allergies.

℘ IRON

Iron helps breastfeeding mothers (and everyone else) maintain their energy level, so be sure to get enough of this important mineral in your diet. Lean meats and dark leafy green vegetables are good sources of iron. Other sources of iron include fish, iron-fortified cereals, and the dark meat in poultry.

When it comes to meeting your iron needs, it's important to eat the best sources of iron and to pair them with the right foods. Iron from animal sources, for instance, is generally better absorbed than iron from plant sources. Tea may interfere with iron absorption, so you may want to avoid drinking tea when you eat iron-rich foods or take iron supplements. On the other hand, foods that are rich in vitamin C can enhance iron absorption. So consider pairing ground beef with spinach, or take your multivitamin/mineral supplement with a glass of orange juice.

℘ FOLIC ACID

Nursing mothers (along with all women of childbearing age) should get at least 400 micrograms of folate, or folic acid, daily to prevent birth defects in future children and ensure their babies' continued normal development. Spinach and other green vegetables are excellent sources of folic acid, as are citrus fruits or juices,

I Don't Eat Meat

SPECIAL DIETS

A special diet is often a healthy diet—in fact, you may maintain a particular diet for health reasons—but it still may not provide all the nutrients you and your baby need while breastfeeding. If your consumption of any major food group is limited, consider how you will replace the missing elements in your diet, *and* discuss your plans with your doctor or nutritionist. Breastfeeding women who do not eat meat, for example, must figure out how they will get sufficient protein for their babies and themselves.

As a vegetarian, you may already be familiar with ways to combine plant foods to meet your needs. You may get protein from rice, beans, eggs, nuts and nut butters, and meat substitutes. If you do not know all the healthy ways to compensate for lack of meat in your diet, consult a registered dietitian. Ask your pediatrician whether you should take a daily vitamin/mineral supplement containing such elements as iron, zinc, and vitamin B_{12}. It is essential that strict vegans (who avoid all animal products in their diet) take a vitamin B_{12} supplement, since this nutrient comes only from animal sources. Keep in mind that you will also need to make sure you consume enough calories to maintain your health—usually between 2,200 and 2,500 per day if you are of average build. If you have any special concerns about your diet, your pediatrician may suggest you consult with a registered dietitian.

many kinds of beans, and meat or poultry liver. You can also get folic acid from breads, cereal, and grains, which are enriched with folate in the United States. All women in their reproductive years are encouraged to take a multivitamin supplement that provides 400 micrograms of folate daily.

∞ A WORD ON SUPPLEMENTS

To make sure you are getting all of the important vitamins and minerals, you may want to continue taking your daily prenatal vitamin or a daily multivitamin. Keep in mind, though, that these supplements are an *addition* to a healthy diet, not a replacement. The fact is, there is no replacement for a daily intake of fresh vitamin- and mineral-rich foods.

WHAT TO AVOID: SUBSTANCES THAT MAY NEGATIVELY AFFECT YOUR BABY

Many women find the need to restrict or alter their diets during pregnancy difficult. It may not be easy for someone accustomed to five cups of coffee a day (or an alcoholic drink or two during dinner) to abruptly change her habits and give up her daily java jolt. After nine months, however, the improvements to your diet and lifestyle may have become routine. If so, you're fortunate: your new, healthier eating habits will help contribute to your baby's health and development—as well as your own health. Still, now that your baby is born, it's natural to wonder whether it's all right to enjoy a cup of coffee with breakfast or a glass of wine with dinner without worrying that doing so will harm your baby.

Fortunately, the mammary glands that produce your milk are able to provide your baby with highly nutritious milk even if your diet isn't perfect every day. As we discussed in Chapter 2, the mammary glands and milk-producing cells also help regulate how much of what you eat and drink actually reaches your baby through your milk.

∞ CAFFEINE

Consuming coffee, tea, and caffeinated sodas in moderation is fine when you are breastfeeding. Breast milk usually contains less than 1 percent of the caffeine ingested by the mom. And if you drink no more than three cups of coffee spread throughout the day, there is little to no caffeine detected in the baby's urine.

However, if you feel that your infant becomes more fussy or irritable when you consume excessive amounts of caffeine (usually more than five caffeinated beverages per day), consider decreasing your intake. Pay attention to the amount of tea and soda you drink and chocolate you eat, too. Most teas, sodas, and chocolate contain caffeine.

∞ ALCOHOL

Alcohol passes through your milk to your baby, so it's best to avoid habitual use while breastfeeding. And while drinking beer does not increase your milk supply, as urban myth suggests, consuming alcohol of any kind may decrease the amount of milk your baby drinks. Alcohol can change the taste of your milk, and this may be objectionable to some babies. If you choose to have an alcoholic drink, it's best to do so just after you nurse or express milk rather than before, and allow at least two hours per drink or two before your next breastfeeding or pumping session. That way, your body will have as much time as possible to rid itself of the alcohol before the next feeding and less will reach your infant.

One alcoholic drink—the equivalent of a 12-ounce beer, 4-ounce glass of wine, or 1 ounce of hard liquor—will probably not harm your baby. However, there are concerns about long-term, repeated exposures of infants to alcohol via the mother's milk, so moderation is definitely advised. Chronic consumption of alcohol may also reduce milk production.

∞ MERCURY

As you know, including fish in your diet is a good way to get protein and healthy omega-3 fatty acids without ingesting too many saturated fats. However, nearly all fish contain some traces of mercury, a metal that occurs naturally in the environment and that is increased by industrial pollution. Most people are not affected by these tiny amounts of mercury. But in babies and small children, mercury can cause damage to the nervous system. That's why women of childbearing age and pregnant and lactating women need to avoid fish that are high in mercury, namely, shark, swordfish, king mackerel, and tilefish. When you do eat fish, it's important to eat varieties that contain less mercury, such as canned light tuna, shrimp, salmon, pollock, and catfish.

Some people may prefer albacore or "white" tuna. But albacore tuna generally contains more mercury than the canned light variety. If you enjoy albacore, limit your intake to 6 ounces a week (about one meal). If you like to eat fish caught in local waters, check local advisories about the safety of the fish. If the information is unavailable, limit your consumption to 6 ounces (about one meal) a week. These same recommendations also apply when you're feeding fish and shellfish to your young child. Just make sure to serve smaller portions.

INFANT ALLERGIES AND FOOD SENSITIVITIES

Human breast milk typically does not cause allergic reactions in breastfeeding infants, but mothers sometimes worry that their babies may be allergic to something that they themselves are eating and passing into their breast milk. In fact, only two or three out of every one hundred babies who are exclusively breastfed demonstrate an allergic reaction—and that's most often to the cow's milk in their mother's diet. In this case, the infant may show signs of severe colic, abdominal discomfort, or a skin rash such as eczema or hives, or may react with vomiting, severe diarrhea (often with blood in the stool), or difficulty breathing that lasts up to several hours after breastfeeding. If you note any of these symptoms, contact your pediatrician right away. While rare—especially among breastfed babies—milk allergies can be severe or fatal. Most babies eventually outgrow their allergy to cow's milk, although food allergies to other substances may be lifelong.

Breastfeeding exclusively for the first six months of life has been shown to significantly lessen the risk and severity of food allergies in families with a strong history of them. Exclusive breastfeeding or breastfeeding in combination with partially or extensively hydrolyzed infant formula also reduces the risk for eczema, a condition of excessively dry and easily irritated skin.

So far, there is no evidence that avoiding certain foods while breastfeeding can help prevent your child from developing allergies or asthma. The exception to that might be eczema: some studies suggest that avoiding certain foods may reduce your baby's risk for developing eczema. Still, if your family has experienced severe food allergies, you might consider limiting your intake of milk and dairy products, fish, eggs, peanuts, and other nuts during pregnancy and while breastfeeding. Monitor your baby carefully for skin rashes, breathing problems, unusual stools, or other allergic symptoms, and be sure to tell your pediatrician about your family's medical history.

∞ FOOD SENSITIVITIES

A few mothers notice minor reactions to other foods in their diet. Some babies cry, fuss, or even nurse more often after their mother has eaten spicy or "gassy" foods (such as cabbage). These reactions differ from allergies in that they cause less-serious symptoms (no rashes or abnormal breathing) and almost always last less than twenty-four hours. If your baby reacts negatively every time you eat a certain type of food and you find this troubling, you can just avoid that particular food temporarily. If these symptoms continue on a daily basis and last for long periods, they may indicate colic rather than food sensitivity. Talk with your pediatrician about this possibility, if eliminating various foods has no effect on your child's symptoms.

BACK IN SHAPE: A NATURAL APPROACH TO LOSING WEIGHT

A popular aspect of breastfeeding is the fact that nursing mothers regain their pre-pregnancy figures more quickly than if they had opted to formula-feed. The breastfeeding process makes use of the fat cells stored in the body during pregnancy. Every day that you breastfeed, your body contributes calories from these fat stores, in addition to the calories from your diet, toward your milk production. This is true even when you increase your diet by the 300 to

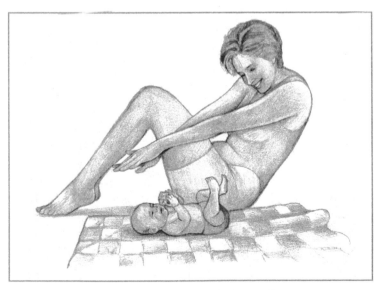

Moderate exercise and a healthy diet can help you regain your pre-pregnancy shape.

500 calories per day recommended to maintain your energy level and ensure adequate milk production. Keep in mind, though, that after an initial loss of about 15 pounds immediately postpartum, the remaining weight loss is more gradual—occurring naturally at about 1 to 2 pounds per month for the first six months after childbirth and somewhat more slowly after that. In most cases, it takes about six to nine months (about the same length of time as your pregnancy) to lose the weight that pregnancy added to your figure.

In the meantime, it is much more important to focus on eating healthy foods than to worry about losing weight. Weight loss methods such as liquid diets, weight loss drugs, or severely cutting calories can negatively affect your milk supply and your baby's health, so avoid them for now. If after six months of breastfeeding you find you need to lose more weight, you can restrict your caloric intake more aggressively after your child has begun to consume solid foods. For now, though, you can regain your figure at a natural, healthy pace by cutting out empty-calorie snacks, substituting skim milk for whole milk, and eating broiled or boiled foods instead of fried ones. Adding moderate exercise is also a healthy way to increase your weight loss.

EATING WELL FOR TWO

No doubt a healthy diet is always important. But it's essential to eat well when you are breastfeeding. Breastfeeding moms need an additional 500 calories a day in the first six months of nursing, which drops to 400 calories in months seven to nine. Make sure to get the extra calories you need from healthy food sources. Nursing moms also need to make sure they are drinking enough fluids. You may notice you're more thirsty than usual when you are breastfeeding. It's often a good idea to drink a glass of water every time you nurse. And remember, a supplement is just that, something that supplements your diet. You should aim to get the bulk of your nutrients from food.

Q & A

Was It Something I Ate?

Q: *I've heard that colicky babies' symptoms can be eased if the mother stops drinking cow's milk. Is this true?*

A: In some cases, colicky symptoms do improve when the mother temporarily avoids cow's milk, even in cases when the infant is not allergic to the milk—perhaps because the infant's digestive system has not yet fully matured. If your baby exhibits such symptoms, discuss with his pediatrician the possibility of abstaining from cow's milk for two weeks, then starting back on milk and observing your infant's response. You will need to continue to have other sources of calcium and vitamin D in your diet if you avoid milk and dairy foods.

Q: *Do the foods a mother eats affect the taste of her milk?*

A: All the foods you eat will flavor your breast milk. In fact, breast-fed infants may be more accepting of new flavors and foods later because they have been exposed to lots of different flavors through human milk. Only in rare cases, however, do babies object to the taste. Even when infants do resist nursing, it is difficult to predict which tastes they will dislike. Generally, your baby may be most likely to enjoy the flavors of foods you enjoyed while pregnant. As with other food sensitivities, this is not an issue to worry about unless it frequently interferes with breastfeeding. In that case, eliminating the unpopular food is a simple solution.

CHAPTER 8

Common Problems:
Solutions and Treatments

One day your baby is nursing like a champ; the next he's turning away from your breast. You're baffled, worried, and anxious. Why isn't your baby nursing when he's obviously hungry? Why does he take a few swallows, then turn away? What did you do differently? Or maybe you have the opposite situation. Your fussy baby suddenly starts nursing voraciously and more frequently, leaving you tired, drained, and concerned. Why is he so hungry? Could it be a growth spurt? How can you keep up with his demands?

The natural process of breastfeeding fluctuates with the changes in you and your baby's moods, experiences, and physical state. Like most nursing mothers, you will soon grow accustomed to your own and your baby's typical responses to such changes and adjust your breastfeeding practices accordingly. You will discover over time that your milk flows more plentifully when you are nursing in a quiet place and feeling calm; that a certain way your baby fusses at the breast may mean he's beginning to get sick and should see his pediatrician; and that tenderness or soreness of your nipples can be cured by switching to a different nursing position.

At times, however, a new situation may surprise you. Your baby may suddenly appear uninterested in nursing or may frantically nuzzle your breast as though he can't get enough to eat. You may worry about passing on an illness that you've contracted. Or you may even find that your body has stopped producing breast milk long before you are ready to wean. If you fear that such situations put your baby's health at risk, or if they cause you physical pain, you will (and should) be especially eager to find solutions as quickly as possible. This chapter covers the most common stumbling blocks to successful breastfeeding. In many cases, the treatments and solutions offered here will be sufficient to help you overcome the problem. If not, however, seek the help of your child's pediatrician or family physician, lactation specialist, or La Leche League volunteer.

WHY DOES IT HURT? TREATING BREAST PAIN

It's not unusual for your baby to have a little trouble latching on the first few times you breastfeed. Some babies suck on the nipple without taking enough of the areola into the mouth, which can result in a lot of pain for you. Your nipples may even become cracked and sore, and you may be tempted to stop breastfeeding.

In Chapter 4, we examined the reasons why your baby's ability to properly latch on to the breast is the essential first step in learning to nurse successfully. In the days and weeks following childbirth, it is important to have your pediatrician or lactation specialist check to make sure that correct latching on has been

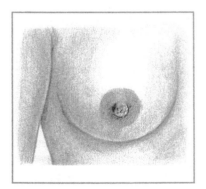

Cracked nipples can be a result of improper latching on.

achieved, since improper latching on can seriously decrease your baby's milk intake as well as your milk production. It can also cause painful cracks in your nipples that will make breastfeeding uncomfortable until they heal.

Many women find that their nipples are somewhat sensitive for the first few days, until they become used to breastfeeding. To prevent soreness, wash your breasts with warm water when bathing and avoid using soap, which can dry and irritate your nipples. If your nipples do become sore or even cracked, check again to be sure that your baby's lips and gums are on the areola as she nurses and not just on the nipple. If possible, vary her position at each feeding. Sometimes a simple switch in positions can make all the difference. Avoid exposing your nipples to excessive moisture between feedings, too. If you are wearing plastic breast shells to treat inverted nipples, remove them after thirty minutes, since these devices hold in moisture. Refrain from using plastic-lined nursing pads for the same reason. Gently pat your nipples dry after a feeding and then apply colostrum, breast milk, or medical-grade purified lanolin to soothe and heal them. (Creams and lotions generally will not help and may actually make the problem worse.) If these steps fail to solve the problem, ask your doctor or lactation specialist for help. In most cases, nipple soreness is a temporary issue and should not stand in the way of successful breastfeeding.

∞ CLOGGED MILK DUCTS

Sometime during the course of breastfeeding, you may experience a sore breast or notice a small lump on your breast that may be red or irritated and hurts when you touch it. This lump may be the result of a clogged milk duct, which can happen if there's an abrupt change in the feeding schedule, inadequate draining of the breast, not varying nursing positions, or wearing clothes or bras that are too tight. A clogged duct should be dealt with immediately since it can lead to a breast infection. The best initial treatment for a clogged duct is to continue nursing, taking care to drain the breast as much as possible with each feeding. (If you suddenly stop breastfeeding, your breast will probably become engorged, which could make the condition worse and lead to an infection.) Before each feeding, gently massage the breast, beginning on the outside and working your way toward the nipple, paying particular attention to the firm area. Breastfeed as often and as long as possible, offering your baby the sore breast first if you can tolerate it, because your baby will nurse most vigorously on the first breast, thus draining it more effectively. Try switching positions to allow better drainage. Express milk from that breast after each feeding if your baby has not completely relieved breast fullness. Apply comfortably warm, moist towels on the affected breast several times a day (or take several warm baths or showers), gently massaging the area around the clogged duct down toward the nipple. If the lump on your breast remains for more than a few days, if it increases in size or redness, or if you develop a fever or significant discomfort, make an appointment to see your doctor.

Keeping pressure off your breasts will help prevent clogged ducts. You can do this by wearing clothing that is not restrictive (avoid tight tops, bras, or underwire bras; if necessary, switch to a larger bra size, or go without a bra for a while); by changing your nursing position so that your baby drains the milk from all areas of the breast equally; and by not sleeping on your stomach. If you notice dried milk plugging the openings in your nipples, wash them gently with warm water after each breastfeeding session. Continued difficulties with clogged ducts may signal a problem with your baby's latching on or with your nursing position. Arrange for a visit with your pediatrician or lactation specialist to correct these problems.

∞ ENGORGEMENT

Your breasts may ache at times when they become uncomfortably full, or engorged. Most mothers have experienced such fullness in their breasts at one time or another as their bodies readjust to a baby's changing demands for breast milk. A little fullness during the first few days after birth is normal, but excessive engorgement, which can occur from missed feedings or a change in how often your baby nurses, can be quite painful. Feeding frequently on demand helps prevent engorgement, but if your baby is nursing as often as she wants and is gaining weight, you may have to take extra measures to relieve the pressure on your breasts. You can, for example, soak a cloth in warm water and put it on your breasts or take a warm shower before feeding your baby. It may also help to express a small amount of milk before breastfeeding, either manually or with a breast pump (see Chapter 9). For severe engorgement, use a cool compress, gel pack, or ice pack between feedings to relieve discomfort and reduce swelling.

Discomfort due to engorgement may also be relieved by feeding your baby in more than one position. Try alternating sitting up, lying down, and using the football hold (see Chapter 4). Gently massage your breasts from under the arm and down toward the nipple to help reduce soreness and promote milk flow. If you have a forceful milk ejection that causes your baby to choke, try feeding her by lying down on your back with her lying on top of you. Take a break in the middle of a session to express a bit more if your baby starts to choke. While you do not want to take any medications without approval from your doctor, acetaminophen or ibuprofen may relieve pain and are safe to take occasionally during breastfeeding. Meanwhile, the best solution for engorgement is to keep breastfeeding. Soon your milk supply will better match your breastfeeding child's demand, and you will feel much more comfortable.

As strange as it might sound, one treatment for engorgement that many breastfeeding women have found effective involves cabbage. Clean, refrigerated cabbage leaves can be either torn into smaller pieces or left whole and applied directly to the breast. Whole leaves will conform to the shape of the breast if the large central stem portion is removed first. Held in place by the bra, the cabbage is left against the breast as desired or until it becomes warm and wilts. The wilted leaves can be replaced by fresh, cool ones. Either green or red cabbage can be used, but red cabbage is more likely to stain a bra or clothing. Many mothers experience an improvement in the pain and swelling of engorgement within hours after using the cabbage. There is limited clinical research on the use of cabbage for engorgement, and the exact way in which cabbage decreases breast swelling is unknown, but the treatment appears to be harmless. For engorgement, cabbage should be used only until the swelling and pain begin to subside. Continued use may decrease the milk supply too much. Some mothers regularly apply cabbage to hasten the resolution of swelling or discomfort that occurs with weaning, especially when weaning occurs over a relatively brief time.

⌒ MASTITIS

When an area of the breast does not drain sufficiently, bacteria may begin to grow in that area and cause an infection, a condition called mastitis. Symptoms of mastitis include swelling, burning, redness, or pain, and you may have fever, flu-like symptoms, or generalized aches. If you have any of these symptoms, let your doctor know at once. Treatment consists of warm compresses and antibiotics, along with frequent breastfeeding, rest, plenty of fluids, and pain medication. When your doctor prescribes antibiotics for mastitis, it is important to complete the entire prescription amount. Many mothers are concerned about the antibiotic being transmitted in the breast milk and affecting the baby, so they either don't take the medicine or stop earlier than recommended. The antibiotics given to treat mastitis do not generally cause any problems for the nursing infant, and failure to complete the course may increase your chance of developing another episode of the infection. Repeat or untreated breast infections may cause scarring, which can impact your milk production even with subsequent pregnancies and breastfeeding experiences.

It's important to continue breastfeeding while you have mastitis, since frequent nursing helps drain your breasts and prevents the infection from spreading. Your baby will not be harmed by drinking your breast milk. Sometimes the breast milk may taste "salty" and may be refused by the baby. If it is too painful to have your baby nurse on the infected breast, move him to the other breast and open up both sides of your bra to let milk flow from the sore breast onto a towel or absorbent cloth. Frequently expressing milk from the affected breast with a breast pump will also help relieve the pressure and speed up the healing process. Milk must be removed from the infected breast either by the baby or with a pump.

CAN HE CATCH IT? MINOR ILLNESSES AND INFECTIONS

Chances are that sometime during the course of breastfeeding you will develop a cold, the flu, a bacterial infection, or other routine illness. In such a situation, you may wonder if the baby will acquire the illness via breastfeeding. Whether breastfeeding or formula-feeding, your infant has been exposed to you and your illness by the time your symptoms develop. Breastfeeding provides added protection and treatment via the milk. It is best to keep breastfeeding, so that the antibodies your body has produced will pass through your milk to protect your baby. If you stop breastfeeding when cold or flu symptoms appear, you actually reduce your baby's protection and increase the chance of his getting sick or having a more severe illness if he does get sick. Even with more serious illnesses—such as gallbladder surgery or a severe infection—you can usually continue breastfeeding or, at most, interrupt feeding for only a brief time. If you are unsure whether a particular illness or infection affects breastfeeding, ask your pediatrician for advice.

One type of infection that may appear among nursing mothers or babies is a yeast or fungal infection. Yeast infections are especially common among women with diabetes and sometimes occur

Expert Help

WHEN TO CALL THE PEDIATRICIAN

Most routine problems that arise during breastfeeding can be easily prevented or quickly cured. There are times, however, when it is vital to have your child examined by his pediatrician without delay. Refusing to breastfeed may be a sign of illness that needs prompt attention. If your baby cannot or will not nurse for any reason, or if you find you are having problems breastfeeding, make an appointment with his pediatrician right away. If your baby continues to feed poorly, your milk supply will begin to decline, so while your baby is being evaluated by his pediatrician, you may need to express your milk.

Other common infant behaviors or conditions that require *immediate* medical attention include extreme fussiness, fever, poor skin color, sleeping through feedings, coughing, or difficulty breathing. Repeated vomiting and reduced urination may also be danger signs. All of these findings are especially worrisome in a young infant.

after a mother or baby has completed a course of antibiotics. Signs of thrush in your baby include milky white spots or a coating on the inside of the mouth. In addition to the spots in the mouth, the baby may have a diaper rash, also caused by the yeast. If the infection is on the mother's nipples, they may appear pink, shiny, oozy, crusty, or flaky, and she may experience a burning sensation in the nipples or breasts during or after nursing, even without other symptoms or signs of the infection.

To prevent thrush, keep your nipples clean and dry. Change your nursing pads when they become damp, and wash your hands often.

Be sure to boil or at least thoroughly wash with warm, soapy water anything that goes into your baby's mouth, including teething rings, pacifiers, artificial nipples, and toys. If you find signs of thrush in your baby's mouth or suspect that you may have a yeast infection of your breasts, contact your doctor and your baby's pediatrician. Always follow the course of treatment prescribed and continue treatment until several days after the symptoms have improved, or the infection may return. Do not rely solely on over-the-counter or home remedies, since these are not likely to completely clear up the infection. It is important for both you and your infant to be treated at the same time, even if only one of you has symptoms. This helps to prevent the infection from spreading back and forth between the two of you. Your doctor might advise you to throw away any breast milk that you expressed and stored while you had thrush, because the yeast can contaminate your breast milk and is not destroyed by freezing. While you are being treated, you can and should continue direct breastfeeding. Though thrush is easily passed back and forth between you and your child (as well as between sexual partners—a possible cause of your infection), stopping nursing will not cure the condition once it has developed.

WHY WON'T HE EAT? COMMON FEEDING PROBLEMS

Feeding problems occur for a number of reasons, many of which vary according to age. In Chapter 4 we described very early impediments to feeding, such as a newborn's sleepiness or difficulty latching on. Most of these challenges can be met through proper breastfeeding instruction from a nurse or lactation specialist and the natural development of a breastfeeding rhythm. It may come as a surprise, then, if your baby develops a resistance to feeding weeks or even months after you thought this was no longer a problem.

One thing to consider when this happens is whether the taste of your breast milk has changed. Breast milk taste can change for a number of reasons, including the following:

- New or different food in your diet
- Medication you are taking
- Pregnancy in the mother, which sometimes causes nursing babies to wean themselves a few weeks or months after the mother conceives
- Strenuous exercise, which can lead to a temporary buildup of lactic acid
- Breast infection, such as mastitis
- Change in the taste of your skin caused by using lotion, cream, or oil on your breasts

Avoiding the new food, changing or stopping your medication if possible, exercising less strenuously, or refraining from applying oil or lotion to your breasts may be all that is necessary to encourage your baby to breastfeed at his normal rate again. If you have mastitis, seek treatment from your doctor right away and encourage your baby to breastfeed in order to drain your breasts. Once the infection has been treated and has passed, the taste of your breast milk will return to normal. You may be able to help your baby adjust to the new taste of your breast milk during pregnancy if you are persistent and patient and hold off on offering formula as an alternative.

If your baby starts to engage in frenzied short feedings that seem to signal frantic hunger, it may simply mean that your letdown reflex is occurring more slowly than she would like. If this is the case, try massaging your breast and expressing a little milk before you begin a feeding. This way, your milk will flow faster from the very beginning of the feeding and your baby will feel more satisfied.

If you do not believe that the taste of your breast milk has been altered or that your let-down reflex is causing the problem, consider whether you are experiencing a high level of tension or stress. Such emotional discomfort can be communicated to your baby, preventing her from settling down to feed well. Of course, we cannot always eradicate stress from our lives, but for the moments preceding breastfeeding, do your best to put upsetting thoughts out of your mind. Relaxed sessions not only will help your baby get more milk but may decrease your own stress level. Breastfeeding your baby and holding her skin to skin often promote a sense of well-being. Meanwhile, consider ways in which you might improve the general tenor of your day-to-day life.

It is also possible that your baby's own condition may be making it harder for her to breastfeed. Decreased interest in feeding—possibly accompanied by lethargy, fever, vomiting or diarrhea, cough, or difficulty breathing—may indicate an illness. Consult your pediatrician or family physician if your baby resists feeding or you have any concerns that your infant may be sick.

Illness in your infant may affect your baby's feeding pattern and desire to nurse, thus decreasing the amount of breast milk she receives. If she has a cold, clogged nostrils may make it difficult for her to breathe while feeding, or an ear infection may make nursing painful. Clearing the infant's nasal passages with a bulb syringe prior to feeding may help with temporary nasal congestion. Teething can cause gum pain when nursing. As pointed out above, thrush can make nursing painful and requires a pediatrician's attention.

Some babies take in a great deal of milk but then spit up what appears to be a large part of it after each feeding. Spitting up is common during or after feeding, and some babies spit up more easily than others. There is generally no need to be concerned, however, that your baby's spitting up is preventing her from getting enough milk. Spitting up (as well as hiccups) can be minimized by keeping your breastfeeding sessions as calm, quiet, and leisurely as possible. Avoid interruptions, sudden noises, bright lights, and other distractions. Try to hold your baby more upright during and right after feedings, and attempt to burp her after she finishes each breast. Don't jostle or play vigorously with her immediately after she has breastfed. If she vomits forcefully a number of times or if you notice blood or a dark green color when she vomits, call your pediatrician right away. Occasional small spit-ups or wet burps are generally more a laundry problem than a medical one. Fortunately, spit-up breast milk is less likely to smell sour or cause clothing to stain than infant formula. If you are worried that she is spitting up too much, consult your pediatrician, who will monitor her weight and check for any signs of more serious illness.

DEHYDRATION

As always, the best way to be sure your baby is getting enough milk is to monitor her physical condition, her weight gain, and the content of her diapers. It is very important to call your pediatrician if you notice that your child is not showing usual interest in feeding, she has a dry mouth or eyes, or she is producing fewer wet diapers than usual. These may be signs of dehydration. Severe dehydration, while uncommon in adequately breastfed infants, can be extremely dangerous or even life-threatening and is most likely to occur when a young baby refuses to feed or is experiencing frequent vomiting or diarrhea.

PROBLEM SOLVED

Fortunately, most difficulties with breastfeeding are temporary and go away with minor interventions. The key is to do some detective work to discover what's causing the problem, whether it might be sore nipples, a clogged milk duct, or a new cold developing in your baby. Once you get beyond the problem and adapt, you can continue breastfeeding your baby with success.

CHAPTER 9

Breastfeeding Beyond Infancy

Months into breastfeeding, you and your baby have forged a tight bond and a healthy rhythm. Some moms have started to abandon nursing, and perhaps you're wondering if you can keep going despite your mother-in-law's disapproving glares and your friends' not-so-subtle remarks. The good news is, the choice is entirely up to you. And if you're not certain, consider this: breastfeeding beyond six months or even a year continues to provide your child with the one-of-a-kind nutritional and emotional benefits that your newborn baby enjoyed.

MORE IS BETTER

It's not uncommon to come up against expressions of surprise or even disapproval as you continue breastfeeding beyond six months or into the second year. Our culture's past history of choosing formula-feeding over the breast has led to confusion over how long it is "normal" for a baby to nurse. Though most people know that mothers in many other countries routinely breastfeed their children into toddlerhood, the sight of an older baby nursing still takes some in the United States by surprise. Even some mothers who have observed the benefits of breastfeeding assume that the first tooth, the first step, or the first taste of solid food is a sign that the time for nursing is over.

Fortunately, this situation is changing. More families are learning of the American Academy of Pediatrics' recommendations that breast milk remain an infant's sole source of nourishment for about the first six months and that breastfeeding continue along with the introduction of solid foods through *at least* the first birthday and beyond for as long as mutually desired by mother and baby. Just as your breast milk provided the perfect feeding for your newborn, so it continues to meet his nutritional, immunologic, and emotional needs as he grows. As he gets older, his relationship with you as a breastfeeding mother will develop, too. He will come to understand, in this quite compelling way, that even as his world expands he can continue to count on you for physical comfort and emotional support. What a wonderful lesson this is for you and your little one to learn!

THE FIRST SIX MONTHS

It is wonderful to know you have triumphed over whatever uncertainties or challenges you experienced during the early weeks of breastfeeding. Now that the two of you have settled into a comfortable relationship, your baby has no doubt become confident about nursing, and the balance between your breast milk supply and your baby's demand has stabilized to some degree. You have probably grown accustomed to her particular style of breastfeeding. You may also have experimented with breastfeeding in public and have a good idea which clothes, positions, and locations work best for you. As time passes, you will find that breastfeeding is a perfectly natural and almost automatic process as you take your child out with increasing frequency. You will be able to anticipate approximately when your baby will want to nurse, respond quickly to her early signs of hunger, and build in extra time for feedings when you are running errands or traveling by car. As you spend more time apart from your child, you'll grow adept at expressing breast milk ahead of time so your baby can be cup- or bottle-fed in your absence.

∞   SUPPLY AND DEMAND: CHANGES IN YOUR
BREASTFEEDING RHYTHM

Growing accustomed to your baby's breastfeeding habits doesn't mean they will never change. As we pointed out in Chapter 6, feedings gradually become less frequent after your baby's first few weeks, falling into a more regular routine of feedings throughout the day and night. Still, for a number of reasons, growing babies may abruptly increase or decrease their demands for feedings, resulting in an unexpected increase or decrease in the number and length of nursing sessions per day. An otherwise regular breastfeeder's sudden insistence on more feedings usually signals a growth spurt—a temporary increase in her rate of growth that requires an increase in calories. A marked increase in activity, such as learning to crawl or walk, may also cause your child to nurse more frequently as she burns up more calories or to nurse less frequently due to her interest in the new activity. Even stress or overactivity in your own life, which can cause your milk supply to decrease, may lead to her acting hungrier and wanting to feed more often.

The best way to respond to such increased demand is to breastfeed more frequently over the course of several days to increase

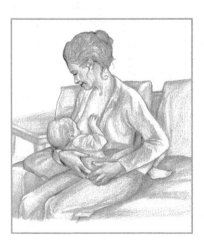

Breastfeeding should be your child's sole source of nourishment for about the first six months of life and should continue along with the introduction of solid foods for at least the first year.

your milk production and satisfy your baby's needs. (During this time, make sure you are getting enough rest and drinking adequate fluids.) Your baby will appreciate the extra feedings, and they will gradually taper off again as her growth rate evens out again, her activity level stabilizes, or your milk supply adjusts. Keep in mind, too, that if the appetite spurt occurs at around six months, your baby may be demonstrating her readiness to begin eating solid foods. As she begins to sample this extra nourishment, she will gradually depend less on your breast milk to supply her with all the calories she needs.

∞ LOSS OF APPETITE

You may find at other times that your older baby has abruptly lost her appetite, feeding for short periods or refusing the breast altogether. In Chapter 8 we discussed reasons that growing babies may lose interest in breastfeeding. In some cases, however, the reason for your baby's decrease in appetite won't be immediately apparent. If you have reviewed and discounted the possible causes for loss of appetite listed in Chapter 8 and have had your baby examined by his pediatrician and his health appears fine, you may simply need to exercise a little patience.

Meanwhile, resist the temptation (or others' urgings) to offer your baby formula or even a bottle of breast milk as a solution to this problem. By using formula, you will decrease your level of milk production even more. By switching to a bottle, you may discourage your baby from returning to the breast when she is ready and able (usually after a couple of days). Better solutions include offering her your breast when she's sleepy and doesn't remember to refuse it; trying new breastfeeding positions that may be more comfortable for her; feeding in a quiet, somewhat dark environment, without distractions from computers, music, or television; and feeding her your expressed breast milk with a spoon, eyedropper, or cup if you are still concerned that she is not breastfeeding enough.

Eventually your baby will probably regain her interest in nursing. If not, it's possible that she is ready to wean or would be happier with some solid foods in her diet. As always, it's best to follow her lead, providing her with the nutrition that best suits her age.

⌒ IS SHE GROWING?

As your child grows, it's important to continue to monitor her weight to be sure she is getting the nutrition she needs. Talk to your pediatrician about interpreting your own child's growth on standard growth curves at her well-child checkups.

If your baby is older than three months and has recently stopped gaining or has even lost weight, consult your pediatrician. Babies at that age should still be gaining weight, even if the rate has slowed a bit. An easily distracted, active, or impatient baby who is not feeding long enough in a session may need to breastfeed in quieter locations and switch breasts frequently in order to stay interested. If you have begun using a pacifier, baby swing, or other device to soothe your baby when she's fretful, try offering your breast instead—thus increasing her number of feeding opportunities. If she is teething (you'll notice her drooling more and perhaps sucking her fist) and thus enjoying her feedings less, make her feeding sessions shorter but more frequent, and give her a one-piece teething ring after each feeding. Again, these are simple solutions for most common problems that temporarily interfere with breastfeeding. If your baby's refusal to breastfeed continues, however, it is vital to have her examined by her pediatrician and to consult with a lactation specialist about maintaining your breast milk supply in the meantime.

Breastfed babies tend to regulate their intake better than formula-fed babies. Breastfed and formula-fed babies seem to grow in a similar fashion for the first three to four months of age. After that time, breastfed babies may seem to grow at a slightly slower, although likely more appropriate, rate. Weight gain that is too rapid may correlate with later incidence of childhood obesity. Though

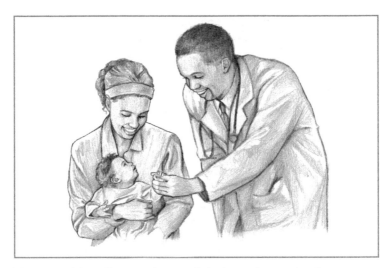

Your pediatrician will ensure that your baby is growing at a steady rate.

too-rapid weight gain is never a problem during the first few months of your breastfed baby's life (a younger baby should always be breastfed on demand), you may start to wonder if your plump older baby is feeding too often. This might be the case for some babies if the breast is offered constantly, even when they have not signaled their hunger. If you do not believe that your baby is hungry, consider exploring with your older baby alternative ways for her to find stimulation or to comfort herself (such as playing peekaboo with her sibling, or rocking in her father's arms). But don't worry too much about excessive weight gain during this first year. The fact is, most breastfed babies regulate their intake of breast milk to meet their needs quite well, and very few breastfed babies are seriously overweight. Your baby probably will start to lose her excess fat as she becomes more physically active after six months of age.

∽   YOUR BABY'S TEETH

Your baby's first tooth probably will appear after six months, though some babies are born with one or more teeth and in other

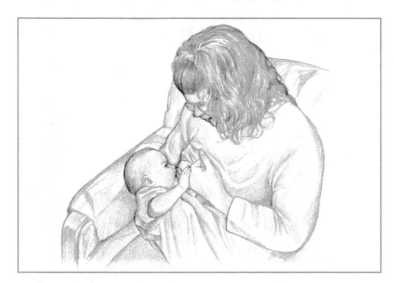

Nursing can continue successfully after your baby develops teeth.

cases teeth don't appear until the child is almost a year old. Many mothers decide that it's time to stop breastfeeding when they first notice a tooth. Usually this is because the baby has nipped the breast at the end of a feeding session or because the mother fears she will be bitten. Yet many babies with teeth (or those who are teething) never bite when breastfeeding. In fact, an actively nursing baby will not bite, because her tongue covers her lower teeth. A baby who nips the breast as he starts to pull away near the end of a feeding can be taught to stop. Try not to let this minor challenge get in the way of breastfeeding so early in your nursing relationship.

If your baby has sprouted a tooth and you are concerned that she may nip you as a feeding ends, keep your finger ready to break the suction and remove your breast as soon as her rhythmic suckling stops (and before she starts to drift off or feel playful). If she has already bitten, say no firmly and then remove her from your breast. Try to keep this action as bland and matter-of-fact as possi-

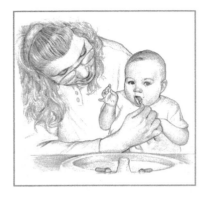

Clean your baby's teeth with a soft-bristled brush after breastfeeding to prevent tooth decay.

ble: too much anger or even amusement may interest her enough to make her want to repeat the experiment again. Once she realizes that biting means no more breast, she will learn to stifle the impulse. (Meanwhile, don't forget to offer her a one-piece teething ring when she is not nursing.)

Once your baby's teeth have begun to come in, it is important to keep in mind that even breastfeeding babies are sometimes susceptible to baby-bottle tooth decay (BBTD), a major cause of dental cavities in infants that can also cause serious damage to permanent teeth later on. BBTD results from teeth being coated in almost any liquid other than water for long periods, and occurs most commonly among babies who are put to bed with a bottle of formula or juice. Research shows that human milk by itself does not promote tooth decay. But breastfeeding infants who fall asleep while nursing with unswallowed milk in their mouths are also vulnerable to tooth decay. Beyond the first year, dental caries—tooth decay—can occur in toddlers who receive sugary liquids in a bottle or who are nursing and also eating foods with sugar and carbohydrates. Make a point of removing your breast from your baby's mouth once she has fallen asleep.

Your pediatrician will check your baby's teeth as part of the well-child visits during the first year of life and beyond. To stimulate healthy gums and good oral hygiene, it is a good idea to wipe the gums at least once a day, beginning at birth, even before any teeth have erupted in your child's mouth. After teeth erupt, wiping her gums and teeth with a piece of gauze or a damp cloth after feedings and before bedtime will help maintain good oral hygiene. Once your child has several teeth, start using water and a soft-bristled, child-sized toothbrush for daily cleaning. Your pediatrician will advise you about when to begin using toothpaste with your child. Fluoridated toothpaste is not usually recommended until after age two, since babies tend to swallow it and can actually get too much fluoride. Some fluoride is good for strong, healthy teeth that are resistant to decay, but too much can cause a permanent, dark discoloration of the teeth. Your doctor or dentist may also apply a topical fluoride varnish at office visits to protect her teeth.

WHEN MOMMY'S AWAY: FEEDING YOUR BABY EXPRESSED MILK

As you become more comfortable with the rhythms and routines of life with your baby, you will no doubt resume activities that were temporarily interrupted by early motherhood. You may need to return to work or want your partner or other caregivers to feed your child occasionally. In such cases, you can use a breast pump to express breast milk that your baby's caregiver can then feed to him in a bottle or cup. This is preferable to offering your baby formula, since infant formula fails to provide him with all the nutrients of breast milk. Infant formula may also decrease breast milk's immune-system-enhancing benefits, puts some babies at risk of an allergic reaction, and may decrease your milk supply if you don't express your breast milk.

An ideal time to introduce your baby to expressed breast milk fed from a bottle is during his second month of life. Before about three or four weeks of age, using a bottle may cause him to refuse the breast—a situation called *nipple confusion*. After age four weeks, he will be settled securely into his breastfeeding habit yet still be open to new feeding experiences. By occasionally letting him drink breast milk from a bottle—even if you will not need to do so regularly until months later—you can teach him to switch easily from bottle to breast and back again. (This advance preparation is not absolutely necessary, however, since almost all breastfed babies can learn to adapt to alternative ways of being fed when the time comes. In most cases, they can adjust within about a week.)

∽ EXPRESSING MILK

Some women are apprehensive about the prospect of learning to express breast milk. Like any skill, though, expressing milk gets easier each time you practice it. Milk can be expressed by hand, with a manual pump, or with a battery-operated or electric breast pump. Though hand-expressing can be challenging for some women to learn, it is the most convenient first choice, because

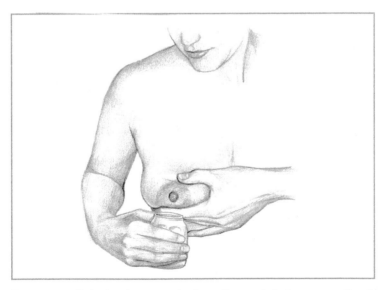

To express milk by hand, press and release the areola between your thumb and fingers with a rhythmic motion.

there is no need for extra equipment (and, of course, it costs nothing). You might want to try this first during a regular breastfeeding, after you have already experienced a let-down reflex. You can express milk from the second breast immediately after a feeding with the first, or even during that first feeding if your partner or someone else can help you. Some women find that expressing milk when they wake up in the morning is easiest, since their milk is more abundant then.

To express by hand, first be sure that your hands and fingernails (preferably short) are clean by washing them with soap and water. (You might even take a warm shower just before expressing, or place a clean, warm, moist towel over your breasts to help you relax and encourage the milk to let down.) Then massage your breast slowly, starting at the outer areas and working your way down toward the nipple. The massage should be gentle, never uncomfortable to your breasts or your skin.

Next, place a clean cup or jar beneath the nipple so that the milk will drip directly into it without touching your hands or your breast. Position your hand on the areola with the thumb above and two fingers below, about an inch behind the nipple. Press back toward your chest, then gently press the areola between your thumb and fingers and release with a rhythmic motion until the milk flows or squirts out. Rotate your thumb and fingers around the areola to get milk from several positions. Avoid squeezing the nipple or sliding down the breast, since this can cause bruising.

Transfer the milk into clean, covered containers for storage in the refrigerator or freezer (see more information on pages 171–172 on storing expressed human milk). If you don't collect any milk this time, try again later—but be aware that your let-down reflex may take a while to occur, and it may then take up to half an hour at first to sufficiently relieve both breasts. With practice, you will probably be able to shorten this time considerably and the amount of milk you collect will increase from perhaps 1 ounce per session to a full bottle or more.

∞   BREAST PUMPS

You may find it easier to express milk with the help of a breast pump. One manual (or hand) pump is the *cylinder type,* which consists of two cylinders, one inside the other. To express milk, you move the outer cylinder back and forth, creating a suction action. The milk collects in the inner cylinder (a plastic jar attached to the pump), which can be used as a bottle. Another type of hand-operated pump, called the *trigger type,* is shaped like a gun with a small jar for collecting the milk. This pump is operated by placing it against the nipple and pulling a trigger, which creates suction. The *bulb-type* manual pump, which looks like an old-style bicycle horn, is not recommended, since the suction created is not usually effective and the device is hard to clean.

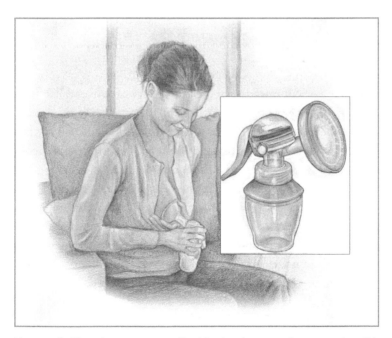

You may find it easier to express milk with a hand-operated pump, such as this trigger-type breast pump.

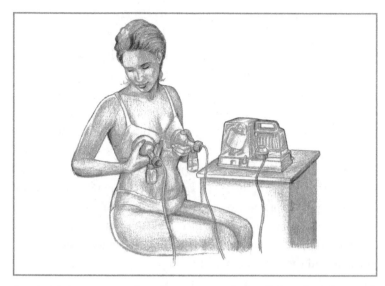

An electric breast pump that allows you to collect milk from both breasts simultaneously is best for mothers who express milk on a routine basis, especially if they have a hospitalized infant.

Small battery-operated or electric pumps are also available for women who express breast milk only on occasion. Full-time working mothers and those who have premature, ill, or physically impaired babies and will be using a pump on a routine basis should use hospital-grade electric breast pumps. A pump with tubing and collection containers that allows you to express the milk from both breasts at the same time works best for this purpose. It's a good idea to talk with your physician or lactation specialist about what type and brand would be most appropriate before you buy. Many types of pumps can be rented instead of purchased, and there's no point in paying for a more expensive pump than you need.

∞   INTRODUCING THE BOTTLE

Once you have learned how to express your breast milk, you will need to teach your baby to drink it from a bottle. Many mothers

Frozen Food

HOW TO STORE AND PREPARE YOUR EXPRESSED MILK

Follow these safe storage and preparation tips to keep your expressed milk healthy for your baby:

- Wash your hands before expressing or handling your milk.
- Be sure to use only clean containers to store expressed milk. Try to use screw-cap bottles, hard plastic cups with tight caps, or special heavy nursing bags that can be used to feed your baby. *Do not use ordinary plastic storage bags or formula bottle bags, since these can easily split and leak.* Do not store breast milk in ice cube trays.
- For a normal, healthy infant at home, use sealed and chilled milk within twenty-four hours if possible. Discard all milk that has been refrigerated for more than ninety-six hours. For infants who are hospitalized, follow hospital guidelines for human milk storage.
- Freeze milk if you do not plan to use it within twenty-four hours. Frozen milk is good for at least one month in a freezer attached to a refrigerator or for three to six months if kept in a deep freezer at 0°F or below. Store it in the back of the freezer, where the temperature is coldest, not in the door. Also, keep the freezer full to maintain lowest temperatures. Be sure to label the milk with the date and time that you expressed it. Use the oldest milk first. Keep in mind that the fats in human milk begin to break down with storage, so using frozen breast milk within three months is desirable.
- Freeze about 2 to 4 ounces of milk per container, to avoid wasting milk after you thaw it. You can always thaw an extra bag if needed.

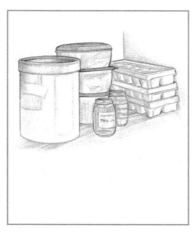

Freeze bottles of expressed milk for later use. Milk is good for at least one month in freezers attached to refrigerators and three to six months in deep freezers at 0°F or below.

- Do not add fresh milk to already frozen milk in a storage container.
- You may thaw milk in the refrigerator or by placing it in a bowl of warm water.
- Do not use microwave ovens to heat bottles, because they do not heat them evenly. Uneven heating can scald your baby or damage the milk. Bottles can also explode if left in the microwave too long. Excessive heat can destroy important proteins and vitamins in the milk.
- Previously frozen milk that has been thawed in the refrigerator must be used within twenty-four hours or discarded.
- Do not refreeze your milk.
- Do not save unfinished milk from a partially consumed bottle to use at another feeding.

find that this works better if someone else offers the baby the bottle at first, somewhere other than where he usually breastfeeds. (That way, he will have none of the usual cues to start seeking out the breast.) Clearly, this is an excellent time to enlist the aid of your partner or other loved one who has been eager to feed him, or perhaps to invite the baby's future caregiver to start establishing a feeding relationship with him.

During the first few attempts, have this person offer about ½ ounce of breast milk an hour or two after a regular feeding, when your baby is alert and motivated to try this new feeding method but not so hungry that he's upset and frantic. The adult should take care to keep a calm and reassuring manner. A smiling face and soothing voice will help your baby relax. It sometimes helps to drip a little familiar-tasting breast milk on the baby's lips or tongue at first to give him an idea of what you are doing. Then slowly and gently introduce the nipple into his mouth. Your baby should be allowed to explore the nipple with his mouth, not have it forced past his gums. Stop the attempt if he becomes frustrated or if more than ten minutes pass and he hasn't fed. It's better to end on a positive note and try again the next day than to create an association between this new method of feeding and feelings of frustration.

If after a few daily attempts he still refuses to drink from the container you've offered, try changing to a different kind of nipple or from a bottle to a cup. (If your baby uses a pacifier, he may prefer a similar nipple for bottle-feeding. Otherwise, you may have to experiment with several types of nipples until you find one he likes.) Some babies are particular about which feeding method they'll accept, but once they are introduced to one they like, they adjust easily. Your baby may show a preference for a small medicine cup or a sippy cup rather than a bottle, even if he is very young. Be aware of your baby's cues and respond accordingly, but don't give up on any one type of feeding device until you've tried it for several days.

As your baby shows signs of accepting an alternative feeding method, start expressing more milk and occasionally offering the bottle or cup when he acts hungry between feedings. Finally, offer him (or have another adult give him) an occasional full, regular feeding with a cup or bottle at a time of day when eventually you expect to be absent. In this way, you can create a daily pattern that will be familiar to your baby by the time you need to implement it.

BREASTFEEDING FROM SIX TO TWELVE MONTHS

Breastfeeding, like many other aspects of parenting, is a gradual process of increasing independence and self-mastery on your baby's part and a gradual stepping back on yours. You may have already experienced the beginnings of this process during the first half year of life as your baby learned to enjoy drinking expressed breast milk from a bottle or cup and you began to go places without her. Still, the two of you were closely tied to each other in a nutritional sense: your child thrived on your breast milk alone, which provided the nutrients she needed. During the second half of the year, your breast milk will continue to provide the great majority of necessary nutrients as she starts to sample a variety of new foods. Though your baby will no doubt greatly enjoy the introduction of new tastes and textures in her life, her experiences with solid food are still just practice sessions for the future. It's important to make sure she continues getting enough breast milk to meet her nutritional needs.

The American Academy of Pediatrics recommends introducing complementary foods at about six months of age. Parents with food allergies are often advised to avoid foods that commonly cause allergic reactions (such as cow's milk, dairy products, and foods made from peanuts or other nuts). But recent research found that the late introduction of certain foods may actually increase your baby's risk for food allergies and inhaled allergies. You should discuss any concerns with your pediatrician. If no allergies are pres-

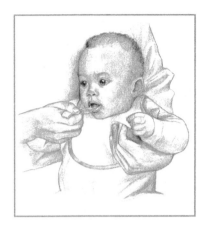

This infant is showing signs of readiness for solid food.

ent, simply observe your baby for indications that she is interested in trying new foods and then start to introduce them gradually, one by one. Signs that the older baby is ready for solids include sitting up with minimal support, showing good head control, trying to grab food off your plate, or turning her head to refuse food when she is not hungry. Your baby may be ready for solids if she continues to act hungry after breastfeeding. The loss of the tongue-thrusting reflex that causes food to be pushed out of her mouth is another indication that she's ready to expand her taste experience.

Since most breastfeeding babies' iron stores begin to diminish at about six months, good first choices for solids are those rich in iron. Current recommendations are that meats, such as turkey, chicken, and beef, should be added as one of the first solids to the breastfed infant's diet. Meats are good sources of high-quality protein, iron, and zinc and provide greater nutritional value than cereals, fruits, or vegetables. Iron-fortified infant cereal (such as rice cereal or oatmeal) is another good solid food to complement breast milk. When first starting infant cereal, check the label to make sure that the cereal is a single-ingredient product—that is, rice cereal or oatmeal—and does not contain added fruit, milk or yogurt solids, or infant formula. This will decrease the likelihood of an allergic reaction with the initial cereal feedings. You can mix the cereal with your breast milk, water, or formula (if you've already intro-duced formula to your baby) until it is a thin consistency. As your baby gets used to the taste and texture, you can gradually make it thicker and increase the amount.

Once your child has grown accustomed to these new tastes, gradually expand her choices with applesauce, pears, peaches, ba-nanas, or other mashed or strained fruit, and such vegetables as cooked carrots, peas, and sweet potatoes. Introduce only one new food at a time and wait several days before you add another new food, to make sure your child does not have a negative reaction. As you learn which foods your baby enjoys and which ones she clearly dislikes, your feeding relationship will grow beyond nursing to a more complex interaction—not a replacement for breastfeeding, certainly, but an interesting addition to it. Remember to keep ex-posing your baby to a wide variety of foods. Research indicates that some babies need multiple exposures to a new taste before they learn to enjoy it. The breastfed baby has already been experiencing different flavors in the mother's breast milk, based upon her diet, so solid foods often have a familiar taste when introduced to the breastfed baby.

Babies need only a few spoonfuls as they begin solids. Since these first foods are intended as complements and not replace-ments for your breast milk, it's best to offer them after a late-afternoon or evening feeding, when your milk supply is apt to be at its lowest and your baby may still be hungry.

Some pediatricians recommend an iron supplement. If this is the case, be careful to give the exact dose prescribed by your doc-tor. Always store iron and vitamin preparations out of the reach of young children in the household, since overdoses can be toxic.

You may find that the number of breastfeedings will gradually decrease as her consumption of solid food increases. A baby who nursed every two to three hours during early infancy may enjoy three or four meals of breast milk per day (along with several snacks) by her twelfth month. Unless you intend to wean her soon, be sure to continue breastfeeding whenever she desires, to ensure your continuing milk supply. To ease breast discomfort, it may become necessary to express a small amount of milk manually on occasion, if her decreasing demand leaves you with an oversupply. Breast comfort is another reason why a gradual introduction of solid foods is advisable, since it allows your body time to adapt to changing demands. Over the span of several months, a readjustment in the supply-and-demand relationship can take place smoothly and painlessly.

BREASTFEEDING BEYOND THE FIRST YEAR

If you are still breastfeeding your child through his first birthday, you can congratulate yourself on having provided him with the best nutrition he could possibly receive. Now that he is consuming a wide variety of solid foods, your breast milk has become somewhat less critical from a nutritional perspective. Some toddlers continue to consume a moderate amount of breast milk (and thus the nutrients it contains), while others "graze" and ingest smaller quantities, getting most of their nutrition elsewhere. Certainly there is no known point at which breast milk becomes nutritionally negligible. What we do know is that as your child moves from babyhood toward toddlerhood, breastfeeding continues to act as a source of profound comfort and security, laying the groundwork for a confident, happy, and healthy future. For this reason, as well as the continued nutritional and immunologic benefits of breastfeeding, the AAP advises mothers to continue nursing beyond the first year for as long as mutually desired by mother and child.

⚮   STARTING THE JOURNEY TOWARD SELF-MANAGEMENT

Many mothers appreciate the power and practicality of breastfeeding to soothe a toddler's emotions, reassure him of their presence, and provide comfort in an often confusing world. Other women worry that continuing breastfeeding into toddlerhood prevents a child from learning to handle his emotions in alternative ways. The fact is, though, that toddlers need emotional reassurance frequently during the day. It is as valid and acceptable for a toddler to breastfeed for comfort as it is for him to suck a pacifier or thumb.

ᴄᴏ DEALING WITH OTHERS' OPINIONS

Our culture can sometimes project a somewhat limited view of acceptable breastfeeding practices; while nursing toddlers are becoming a more common sight, they still occasionally provoke comments and stares from uninformed adults. When deciding how long to breastfeed your child, a more valid yardstick than public opinion is your own child's approach to nursing and your own feelings about it. These feelings are no doubt being communicated to your child. Do you feel that he is dependent on the breast for comfort to the point that it interferes with his social growth (just as a toddler whose relationship with his blanket is so intense that he's unable to put it down to play with a friend)? Are you concerned that his continued nursing is causing other adults (such as a child care provider, preschool teacher, or other important person in his life) to label him in negative ways? Are your own mixed feelings about breastfeeding a toddler interfering with your relationship with him, making you a reluctant and less supportive partner? If your answers to all of these questions are no, then there is no reason to hasten the weaning process.

Mothers who have chosen to continue breastfeeding their toddlers have found many creative ways of dealing with the surprise and uninformed disapproval they encounter among other adults. Many women teach their children a "code word" to use when they want to breastfeed (such as "mimi" or "nonny"), so that the matter remains private between the two of them. Some women then retire with their toddlers to a private place to breastfeed. On the other hand, others make a point of breastfeeding in public, perhaps in the hopes of making it more acceptable for toddlers to continue nursing.

Certainly even in this country the general attitude toward breastfeeding is gradually improving. Thanks to political activism by parents' groups and professional organizations, many states have enacted laws protecting a woman's right to breastfeed. In fact, as of 2010, forty-four states, plus the District of Columbia and the Virgin Islands, had laws allowing mothers to nurse in any public or private location. Only five states have no breastfeeding laws of any kind. Most of these laws state that it is a woman's right to breast-feed wherever she can legally be with her baby. Federal legislation guarantees the right of breastfeeding mothers to nurse their babies anywhere on federal property where the mother and baby have the right to be. This is a good thing not only for mothers, who so frequently have been harassed simply for caring for their children, but also for children, who benefit from all the nutrition, comfort, and love they receive. There is even federal legislation to protect the rights of working mothers to express their milk at the workplace.

My Turn!

NURSING YOUR TODDLER DURING PREGNANCY AND NEW MOTHERHOOD

Women who become pregnant while breastfeeding an older child often wonder whether they can continue nursing through pregnancy and after the new baby's birth. The answer is a qualified yes to both questions, depending on your medical history, your older baby's responses, your own feelings, and your milk supply. Breastfeeding mothers who have miscarried previously or who have a history of premature delivery should stay in touch with their obstetrician and report any uterine contractions, since the nipple stimulation of breastfeeding may increase your risk of delivering too soon. Most often there is no cause for great concern, but it's important to be sensitive to your body's signals. After the first few months of pregnancy, your milk supply will probably diminish somewhat, and the taste of your breast milk may change as well. Either of these changes may cause your baby to refuse the breast milk and eventually wean himself. You may initiate weaning yourself if you experience too much nipple tenderness or physical discomfort. If you and your older baby do continue breastfeeding, it is important to keep in mind that pregnancy and breast milk production both require extra energy. Be sure to monitor your food intake as you prepare for childbirth and get plenty of rest.

Breastfeeding both your older child and your infant, called *tandem nursing*, can in some cases ease your older child's adjustment to the new baby, address your own desire to maintain closeness with the older child, and even make child care easier in some cases as both children are fed and comforted on the breast. Again, though, tandem breastfeeding takes more energy than nursing a single child. Keep in mind that the new baby's breastfeeding needs are the most important at this time. Your infant urgently needs the colostrum (your milk composition will return to colostrum with the birth of your new child and will progress through the stages of milk as defined in Chapter 2) and immune-protective benefits more than your older child. To ensure that your infant receives adequate milk, breastfeed her before nursing your older child and allow her breastfeeding needs to take top priority. A one-year-old or toddler can make up for a decrease in breast milk with nutritious solid foods. When taking care of a newborn or young infant and older children as well, be sure to wash your hands frequently to prevent germs passing from one child to another.

WE'RE DOING FINE, THANKS: DECIDING WHAT'S BEST FOR YOUR CHILD

In the end, the decision about how long to breastfeed your baby is one that only you—with help from your baby—should make. The nursing relationship is a unique bond, one that ideally should be supported by your partner and other family members. So whether it ends when your baby is six months old or three years old is a personal choice. Follow your instincts, and do what is best for you and your baby.

What Changes Should I Look For?

Q: *I've been breastfeeding exclusively since my baby was born and assumed that I wouldn't get pregnant as long as that continued. Now that my baby is six months old, he's begun to eat a little cereal in addition to breastfeeding. Can I get pregnant now that my baby isn't breastfeeding exclusively?*

A: As we pointed out in Chapter 6, breastfeeding is a reliable form of contraception if you are exclusively breastfeeding, if your menstrual periods have not resumed, and if your baby is less than six months old. Once your baby is six months old and has begun sampling solid foods, breastfeeding is no longer a reliable form of birth control. If you do not want to become pregnant, you need to consider what kind of contraception you will use. It's best to consult your gynecologist for advice on which types to use while breastfeeding, but in general, condoms, a diaphragm, or a cervical cap and spermicide are considered the most preferable forms of birth control for a breastfeeding mother, because they are least likely to interfere with the milk supply. Low-dose birth control pills should not have a significant impact on your milk supply when begun at this stage. Injectable hormones, such as Depo-Provera, may be used after the milk supply is well established.

Q: *I started introducing my nine-month-old to solid foods several months ago. Lately there has been some strange-looking red stringy stuff in his diaper. Should I take him to his pediatrician?*

A: As your baby experiences a variety of new foods, his bowel movements will look quite different from the yellowish, curd-like stool of an exclusively breastfed infant. It will begin to resemble and smell more like an adult's stool. You can expect occasional undigested or poorly digested elements to appear in his diaper. Babies don't really chew foods. They gum them and then swallow them, so when they start to eat small soft pieces of fruits and vegetables, you may see these in the stool. You can also expect a change in the frequency of stools after solids are added to the infant's diet. All of these are normal developments, but if you become concerned, call your child's pediatrician.

Q: *Is it okay to give my breastfeeding baby fruit juice every once in a while?*

A: After six months, you can offer your child small amounts of 100 percent fruit juice fortified with vitamin C now and then—as long as the juice serves as an addition to, not a replacement for, her usual intake of breast milk. Juice provides only a tiny fraction of the nutrients found in breast milk; if your baby fills up on juice, she may actually become malnourished. For babies and toddlers, the AAP recommends no more than 4 to 6 ounces of juice per day.

Q: *I taught my baby to drink from a cup at age nine months, and within a few weeks he had completely lost interest in breastfeeding. Did I do something wrong?*

A: Some babies do lose interest in breastfeeding between nine and twelve months of age, whether or not they learn to drink from a cup. Understand that he is not rejecting you; it's just the first sign of your child's growing independence. If you wish, you can continue to express your breast milk for him to drink from a cup. His desire to feed himself "like a big boy" doesn't mean he has to give up the valuable nutrients you provide. He may still enjoy an early-morning or late-night breastfeeding session even after he has stopped nursing during the day.

CHAPTER 10

When You and Your Baby Are Apart

During the first three months of your baby's life, you and your infant have developed a comfortable routine that is both joyful and busy. Now, with your maternity leave drawing to an end, you may be wondering how you and your baby will fare during your transition back to work. You're certainly not ready to stop breastfeeding your baby, and your baby continues to derive important nutrients from your milk. But you wonder if you'll really find the privacy, time, energy, and support to maintain your milk supply.

Most women who plan to continue breastfeeding while working or attending school outside the home worry about how much support they will receive from their employer and co-workers or teachers and administration, and whether they will find the time and energy to accomplish their goal. The advantages are clear: by expressing milk at work or school, mothers feel more connected to their babies and are able to continue breastfeeding during non-working hours. Companies find that breastfeeding women spend less time absent due to their infant's illnesses. Nursing moms are also more satisfied employees who are likely to remain loyal to and working for the company. Still, the idea of combining work and breastfeeding is not a familiar one for many employers. If you intend to continue breastfeeding, it's necessary to prepare your employer, your baby, and yourself ahead of time, assemble a strong support team, and maintain optimism through whatever temporary challenges may arise.

HOW WILL I BREASTFEED AFTER I RETURN TO WORK?

Ideally, preparation for your return to work as a breastfeeding mother should begin long before you have your baby. While you are still pregnant, ask your supervisor or your company's human resources department for information on the company's policies and history regarding all issues relating to a breastfeeding employee's return to work. Ideally, this may include any or all of the following: flexible work schedules, extended maternity leave, on-site child care (so the mother can make frequent short visits to breastfeed), bringing the baby to the office to breastfeed, and provisions for a private place and regular breaks for expressing milk for later use.

As part of the federal Patient Protection and Affordable Care Act of 2010, section 4207 says that employers with fifty employees or more must provide nursing mothers with "reasonable break time" and a private space that isn't a bathroom to pump milk until the employee's baby is twelve months old. Companies with fewer than fifty employees are also supposed to comply with the law unless they can show that doing so would cause undue hardship or expense.

In addition, many states have passed laws protecting the rights of breastfeeding women in the workplace. In New York, for example, companies are legally mandated to provide mothers with a place and time to breastfeed or express milk for their babies. Elsewhere, an increasing number of employers voluntarily provide private rooms for breastfeeding mothers and even allow the baby to be brought to the work site to nurse. Larger corporations may provide one or more breast pumps on-site for all their breastfeeding employees—selling or giving each such employee a personal kit that connects to the pump. In some cases, a lactation specialist is provided to answer questions and help employees learn how to use the pump and maintain their milk supply while back on the job. In short, you may be surprised at what options are available to you. Talk with other mothers at your company about what they have been able to arrange. If not much has been provided for breastfeeding workers in the past, perhaps you and any other concerned employees can volunteer to help establish these lactation support services.

In other cases, no provision at all has been made previously for mothers to breastfeed or to express milk for their babies while on the job. If this is your situation, you will need to talk with your supervisor about your needs and make sure that your employer is aware of the legislation to provide you the protection to express your milk. Such a discussion may be more successful if you come to the meeting with most of the solutions already figured out. Scout out a private, preferably quiet place where you would be able to breastfeed or use a breast pump to express milk. The ideal location for expressing milk would have a sink for washing hands and breastpump parts, a comfortable chair with a table or desk to use for pumping, an electrical outlet, a refrigerator for storing the milk

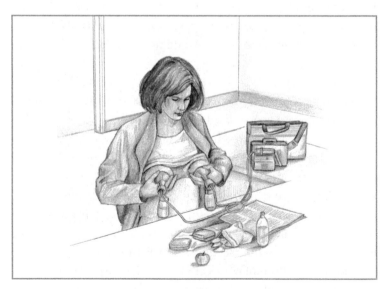

A private office with a door or a designated lactation room is ideal for mothers who wish to express milk at work.

during the daytime, and a lock on the door. (You will also need a portable cooler—the kind with a shoulder strap works best—with ice packs to keep the milk chilled as you carry it home.)

Of course, many women express milk or breastfeed at work in less-than-ideal situations. If you have a private office, you can install a half-size or quarter-size compact (dormitory-type) refrigerator, available for sale or rent at relatively low cost, and wash your hands and pump parts in the ladies' room. (After work, take the pump parts home to be cleaned.) Many women obtain permission to install a table, chair, and refrigerator in a storage closet or other unused space, and they hang a *Privacy Please* sign on the doorknob if the door has no lock. If you do not have access to a refrigerator, you can store your milk in a small portable cooler with ice packs. Be sure to place the milk in the refrigerator or freezer as soon as you return home.

You must also consider how you can schedule time for pumping or breastfeeding sessions during the workday. You'll probably need to express milk every three to four hours, around the times that your baby would normally breastfeed. Each session will last about fifteen to twenty minutes, though you should plan for slightly more time at first while you are adjusting to this new situation (the less time pressure you feel while pumping, the easier your milk expression is likely to be). Your traditional employee breaks and part of your lunchtime may provide you with the time you need. If not, you will have to ask for a little extra time, volunteering to make up that time in the morning or at the end of the day. If you foresee any potential scheduling problems or conflicts with other employees, come up with solutions ahead of time and enlist your co-workers' support. The idea is to demonstrate to the people who work with you that as a nursing mother, you will maintain your standard work productivity. As long as others are reassured about this, they will be more likely to accommodate your needs during this time.

When you meet with your supervisor, lay out your plans simply and clearly. Describe any agreements you have made with co-workers about break times. If you know of other women who have pumped or expressed milk or breastfed at your company, refer to their experience to demonstrate that your solutions and concerns are sound. You might also provide information on the advantages of breastfeeding for mother, baby, and business obtained from the United States Breastfeeding Committee, the American Academy of Pediatrics, or La Leche League websites (see Appendix 1). Most mothers find that their employers are willing to provide both a private space and use of break time. Once you and your supervisor have worked out the logistics of your breastfeeding plan, write them down in memo form and ask your supervisor to initial it and give you a copy. This will prevent any confusion or conflicts when you return to work.

Housed within the National Women's Health Information Center (www.womenshealth.gov) is a program called the Business Case for Breastfeeding aimed at educating employers on the benefits of providing support to nursing mothers in the workplace. The Business Case for Breastfeeding website has information for both workers and employers on creating a lactation-friendly workplace as well as resources for support in the community. It also provides facts and figures on the economic benefits to the company, or "return on investment." These include:

- One-day absences to care for an ill child occur more than twice as often for women who formula-feed their infants compared to those who breastfeed.
- Companies with lactation support programs had an employee retention rate of 94.2 percent. Companies without lactation support programs had a retention rate of 59 percent.
- For every $1 spent by the company on a comprehensive lactation program, the company saved $3.

The materials produced to support the Business Case for Breastfeeding are available online. Through federal grants, most states have offered comprehensive training in promoting the Business Case for Breastfeeding to employers.

∞ AFTER YOUR BABY IS BORN

Even if you did not prepare for breastfeeding before your maternity leave, it is still possible to get ready before your return. Make an appointment with your supervisor to discuss the topics outlined above. During this discussion, reaffirm your desire to perform well at your job and point out that organizing a place and predictable times for milk expression will help you maintain work efficiency. If you meet with resistance, consider ways to schedule breastfeeding sessions on your own during lunch, during scheduled coffee breaks, and before and after work—in your locked office, an unused room you have located, or even the ladies' lounge if necessary. Expressing milk in the restroom is the least desirable location, due to lack of privacy, concerns about sanitation, and aesthetically unpleasing surroundings, so this is no longer recommended.

If you are threatened with the loss of your job because you are expressing milk, you can pursue several options. First discuss the situation with your supervisor, another superior, or someone from the human-resources department. At the same time, gather information and support from your physician, lactation specialists, or the La Leche League (see Chapter 3) and consider speaking with an experienced attorney. Be aware of the Department of Labor regulations to support the Patient Protection and Affordable Care Act of 2010, and keep in mind that it's much better to try to settle any conflicts in a reasonable way rather than face the expense of a lawsuit. In many cases, your own positive, can-do attitude, bolstered by the knowledge that medical opinion supports your efforts, will deflect negative attitudes.

∞ RETURNING TO SCHOOL

Mothers who plan to attend school or college while continuing to breastfeed can use methods similar to those of working mothers.

Discuss your intention to continue breastfeeding with your guidance counselor, a trusted teacher, the dean of women, or another appropriate member of the administration. Find out whether on-site child care is provided at your institution. (If it isn't and you are

A Time for Everything

ALTERING YOUR SCHEDULE TO ACCOMMODATE YOUR BABY'S NEEDS

One way to successfully combine a job or school with breastfeeding is to change your schedule to accommodate nursing, if your personal circumstances permit. By extending your maternity leave, you will have more time to establish a breastfeeding routine. The longer you can stay with your baby full-time the better, so request as much time as possible. You might also explore the possibility of working from home one or two days per week—or even full-time—while you are still nursing. Perhaps you could start back to work or school part-time and gradually increase your hours as the weeks or months pass. (Mothers who work part-time are likely to breastfeed longer than those who work full-time.) Some breastfeeding women even share their jobs with another worker, giving them more time at home. Don't assume that your supervisor will refuse requests of this kind. Many employers understand that offering support to a breastfeeding employee offers long-term benefits to the company, raises morale (improves employee retention), and decreases retraining costs. You may discover that other women at your workplace have already enjoyed such benefits. Unless you ask, you might miss out on just the arrangement that would work best for you and your child.

attending high school, ask your counselor whether there is another school in your area that does offer child care and other services for students with children. Your counselor may also be able to steer you toward parenting courses and La Leche League groups that can further support your efforts to breastfeed while attending school.) Ask for help in finding or creating a suitable place for milk expression—for you and any other breastfeeding students. Again, it is better to approach the administrator with a proposal already in mind than to expect others to make the effort to find space and time for you. If you can provide a clear, easy-to-implement breast-

What Would You Do If . . .

ISSUES TO DISCUSS WITH A POTENTIAL CAREGIVER

No parent wants to change caregivers once a relationship has been established. To ensure that your caregiver is the right choice for you and your baby—and that she will help you maintain your breastfeeding relationship with your child as you return to work—discuss the following issues with her ahead of time:

- Her willingness to feed your baby expressed milk
- How to handle and store your milk
- How your baby prefers to be held for a bottle-feeding
- How to cope with resistance to the bottle
- How to comfort your baby when he's upset
- Whether she feels comfortable delaying a bottle-feeding if you'll arrive soon and can breastfeed
- What to do if you're late picking up your baby
- Your baby's eating, sleeping, elimination, and behavior patterns

feeding plan, your transition to life as a mother-student should be a smooth one.

∽ SELECTING A CAREGIVER

Once you have a good idea what to expect from your employer, it's time to consider who will care for your baby while you work. If you can arrange for child care at or near your office, you may be able to breastfeed even after you return to your job by visiting your baby during breaks. Whether you plan to breastfeed during work hours or have the caregiver feed your milk to your baby, be sure to select a caregiver or child care program that supports breastfeeding and will follow your instructions for handling and feeding of your milk. Discuss such topics as what to do about your baby's resistance to a cup or bottle, whether to delay a feeding if you are due to arrive soon, and so on (see box on page 191); be sure that your philosophy melds easily with the caregiver's intentions or the center's policies. At least once before you start back to work, leave your baby with the caregiver for a period of several hours that includes a feeding. In this way you can work out some of the kinks in the system that might otherwise prove discouraging later.

A MANAGEABLE COMBINATION: BREAST, PUMP, AND BOTTLE

Now that you have prepared your employer for your reentry into the workplace, it's time to prepare yourself and your baby. In Chapter 9 you learned how to hand-express or use a manual or battery-operated pump to express milk for your occasional absences. For mothers who work regularly outside the home, however, a quality hospital-grade electric breast pump is much more efficient and effective. A pump with connections that allow you to express milk from both breasts at the same time is best, since you will generally collect more milk in less time. This type of pump is also most helpful for maintaining a good milk supply. Electric breast pumps can be rented from your hospital or a medical-supply store, or you can buy one (see Appendix 1). Make sure that all parts of the pump that come into contact with your skin or milk can be removed and cleaned. Otherwise, the pump can become a breeding ground for bacteria, and the milk will not be safe for your baby. Some mothers find that keeping a set of clean, duplicate parts at the office saves them a great deal of worry and comes in handy on days when they realize they forgot to wash out the pump attachments the night before.

At first you may not find it easy to use an electric breast pump on both breasts at once, but with practice you will soon master the technique. The best time to practice is after a morning breastfeeding session, when you are likely to have a surplus of milk and your let-down reflex has already occurred. Beginning at least two weeks before you start back to work, try to express milk at least once each day if possible, freezing the breast milk for future use (see Chapter 9 for information on safely handling and storing breast milk). Stockpile as much breast milk as you can— at least enough to feed your baby on your first few days back at work and to allow for the unexpected (spills, missed pumping time at work, a sudden increase in your baby's consumption) during the first few weeks. Regularly pumping and freezing your surplus milk not only will keep your milk production high but also will condition your body to respond to the pumping sensation with a milk ejection reflex. Many mothers find that pumping more than once a day during this period adds greatly to their confidence as they prepare to return to work.

In Chapter 9 we explored ways to help your baby adjust to drinking breast milk from a bottle or cup. Starting this process well before your return to work will help ease the transition for both of you, but your baby will probably adjust satisfactorily even if you have only one week to prepare. If you have already chosen a caregiver, these practice feedings would be an excellent way for the two of them to get to know each other. Just remember to wait until your baby is at least three to four weeks old, if at all possible, so that your milk supply is well established.

EXPRESSING MILK ON THE JOB

Readjusting to your previous work routine can be challenging enough without factoring in a breastfeeding schedule. Fortunately, you have taken the time to prepare your baby, your caregiver, your co-workers, and yourself for this new situation, so you are making the transition in the best possible way. Starting back to work in the middle of the workweek will make it easier for everyone to adjust to the change, since this will provide you with a two- or three-day trial period before you take on a full workweek. Plan ahead to take certain items to work with you each day. Many women get everything together the night before. You will need your pump, a cooler for transporting and perhaps storing breast milk, and a lunch or snacks to help keep your energy up. You may also want to wear breast pads and pack a clean blouse or blazer in case of milk leakage or spills.

On the first day back at work, check in with your supervisor; remind him about your agreement regarding your breastfeeding schedule and make sure that the space allocated for expressing milk is still available. (If possible, visit during your maternity leave to check on the space and to finalize any arrangements. This will ease your mind on that busy first day back.) When you begin your first pumping sessions, try to relax and keep your mind off the people waiting for you outside the room. Any stress could delay your let-down reflex or reduce your milk supply, delaying your return even more. Trying to do paperwork or computer work at your desk or making phone calls while pumping is generally not effective. Thinking about your baby—how comforted she will be as she drinks your breast milk and how good for her your milk is—may help you relax and start your milk flow. Some women find that looking at a photograph of their baby or even listening to a tape of her hunger cry works like a charm.

As you adjust to your new routine, you'll learn ways to integrate your pumping schedule into your day. This will become easier as your co-workers grow used to your brief absences one to three times per day and see that you can still be productive in spite of them. You will learn how to slip discreetly out of a meeting that has run long and is interfering with your pumping schedule—just as another co-worker might excuse himself to visit the restroom. You may even find how easy it can be to recover from or laugh at any snafus—a milk stain on a blouse or an interrupted pumping session—with the help of supportive and empathetic friends.

As you continue to express breast milk at work, monitor how much you are producing. Diminished milk supply is a common problem for employed mothers and is most often the result of skipped pumping sessions or not pumping long enough. Also, pumping may not express as much milk as a baby can get from a breastfeeding session if he is an effective nurser. To increase your supply, pump more frequently for at least ten minutes per session, even if your milk stops flowing before then. When at home with your baby, offer him the breast at least every two or three hours. If he sleeps through the night, consider waking him at your bedtime for an additional feeding. On weekends, breastfeed exclusively and nurse whenever he shows an interest. Once your milk production has increased again, maintain your supply by drinking an adequate amount of liquids, getting enough rest, and relaxing as much as possible during pumping sessions. Remember, cutting a session short to get back to work a few minutes earlier isn't worth the cost in terms of your long-term breastfeeding relationship with your baby. If these suggestions don't help, contact your pediatrician or lactation specialist for additional advice.

ALTERING YOUR SCHEDULE

Many women have found that gradually adjusting their breast-feeding schedules at home reduces the need to pump milk during work hours. Some babies are happy to increase their nighttime nursing to make up for one or two missed daytime feedings—eliminating the need for one pumping session per day. (This works especially well for mothers who are comfortable keeping their babies close to them at night—perhaps in a bassinet near their bed—so that they don't have to wake up completely to breastfeed.) Others find that a feeding just before work, a bottle of expressed milk at lunchtime, and another feeding immediately after work is sufficient to get them through the day, especially when their babies are almost six months old. Some women who have well-established milk supplies express more breast milk on weekends than they normally do during the week, and use this to stock up on their supply. This means less pumping at work. As you experiment with variations on your original nursing rhythm, you will find your own best solution to the challenge of supply and demand. *If you do not pump during the workday, or if you go for long periods without pumping, you will notice a gradual decrease in your milk supply over time.*

As your baby begins to sample solid foods and juices after age six months, you may find that you need to express milk at work less frequently. Some women choose to substitute one or more daily breast milk feedings with formula or solids, eliminating the need for one or more pumping sessions at work. If so, plan to make this change gradually to avoid the risk of uncomfortable breast engorgement and an imbalance in your milk supply. Over the course of a week, pump less milk each time during the session to be eliminated, finally just pumping or hand-expressing enough milk to ease discomfort and prevent leaking. Continue to collect and store your breast milk to freeze for possible future use. By the end of the week, you should have adjusted to the decreased number of daily pumpings.

By your child's first birthday, you will probably have stopped pumping at work altogether, simply breastfeeding when you are together and having his child care provider offer him water, milk, or juice when you aren't there. Looking back, you may consider the time you spent pumping surprisingly short—certainly worth the effort when you consider the many months of breastfeeding benefits your baby received as a result.

GETTING THE HOME SUPPORT YOU NEED

No one—especially a new mother—lives in a vacuum, and you will find it easier to combine breastfeeding with work outside the home if you have the support of family, friends, and experts. In fact, lack of such support is one of the most frequently cited reasons that a woman might stop breastfeeding before her baby reaches the age of six months. Your partner can play a vital role by helping your baby adapt to a bottle or cup as you prepare to return to work, by transporting her to and from the caregiver (or caring for your child himself when this is possible), by arranging for a quiet, uninterrupted "reunion time" for you and your baby at the end of the workday, and by reaffirming your decisions to return to work and to continue breastfeeding as you do so. Having your partner help with household responsibilities will allow you more time to either breastfeed at home or rest as you adjust to a busy schedule.

Friends and relatives can lend an ear, share their own related experiences and wisdom, and refer you to helpful groups, programs, and other information sources in your area. Your pediatrician, lactation specialist, and other breastfeeding experts can advise you on which breast pump is most appropriate for your needs, help you master the technique of pumping milk, and suggest ways to ease your baby's adjustment to a new feeding routine. Community breastfeeding support groups for working mothers can offer valuable management tips and reinforce your decision to keep nursing. If you have a caregiver who is supportive of your breastfeeding plan, you will find her help and encouragement invaluable. And don't forget to support yourself during this period by getting enough rest, drinking plenty of liquids, and taking time now and then for yourself.

WORK AND BREASTFEEDING: A HEALTHY ROUTINE

By the time your first business trip or major work event rolls around, you'll have developed a routine that makes breastfeeding possible while working. For starters, you'll most likely have a suitable caregiver by then, and your baby will be eating solid foods and drinking liquids from a cup. Your partner will have learned to make the necessary accommodations in his schedule, too. Maybe one or both of your baby's grandmothers will have stepped in to help as well. Even expressing milk at the office has probably become a breeze by now.

The ability to juggle work responsibilities with breastfeeding is well worth the trouble when you consider the emotional bond you have with your child. For all your effort, you'll be rewarded with a new confidence in your ability to manage your job and take care of your family too.

Q & A

Will I Be Able to Keep Nursing?

Q: *My boss and co-workers are very supportive of my efforts to continue breastfeeding. Oddly enough, though, my husband doesn't see the point of it. Now that we have a freezer full of expressed milk, he constantly suggests that I "just give the baby a bottle" instead of breastfeeding when we're at home. It's easy to get discouraged with the whole process when your family keeps telling you it's not worth the trouble. How can I get him to help?*

A: Your husband may not understand the role that nursing plays in maintaining milk production and may not fully appreciate the closeness and sense of security that breastfeeding promotes in your child. He may even be acting out of unacknowledged jealousy of the baby's central role in your life right now. Be supportive, but also remind him why you prefer to breastfeed, that expressed milk fed with a bottle is a welcome but less desirable substitute for the real thing, and that without frequent nursing your milk supply will soon disappear. Remind him how effectively nursing soothes your baby to sleep. Then spend some time and effort making him feel appreciated, so he feels like part of the family too.

Q: *I prepared carefully for my transition back to work, but in spite of all my efforts my six-month-old has completely lost interest in breastfeeding in the four weeks since I returned to my job. Is there anything I can do about this?*

A: Some babies—particularly those older than six months—do gradually lose interest in breastfeeding as they adapt to the bottle. Frequently this loss of interest is tied to a lower milk supply. To correct it, make a point of breastfeeding your baby frequently and always on demand—to comfort or soothe as well as nourish him. Breastfeed in a quiet, dimly lit place with few distractions, and consider increasing the number of night feedings. If he doesn't complete a breastfeeding session, pump the remaining milk from your breasts to increase your milk supply. Be aware, though, that some older babies simply wean themselves naturally at this point. If your baby has benefited from exclusive breastfeeding until now, congratulate yourself on providing him with the best possible nutrition for as long as he needed it.

CHAPTER 11

The Father's Role *

As the father or non-breastfeeding partner in a family with a newborn, you may be wondering about your place in the family. Your partner provides round-the-clock nourishment, attends to your baby's cries in the middle of the night, and breastfeeds her around the clock to nourish and emotionally support her. If the mother is still at home on maternity leave, she's probably been primary caregiver to your child for several weeks or even months. You're thrilled to have such a devoted and loving mother for your child and you're glad she's made such a committed effort to breastfeed. Sometimes, though, you can't help wondering, *When is it my turn to assume a bigger role in my baby's care? What exactly am I supposed to do?*

AND NOW WE ARE THREE

A great deal of attention has been paid to the new mother's emotional experience as she adjusts to the role of caregiver, but her partner, too, often feels overwhelmed by the elation, exhaustion, wonder, and concern that come with being a new parent. When the mother is breastfeeding, her partner may feel excluded at first as mother and infant focus on the rhythms of nursing, sleep, and comforting. This intense connection is a natural and important

---

*We recognize that there are different family configurations, and the reader is advised that partner may be substituted for father.

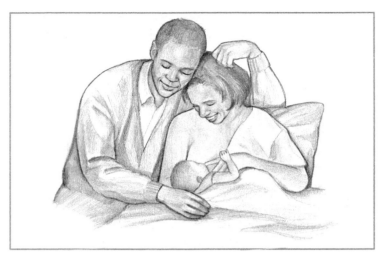

Making breastfeeding a priority gives both parents a chance to spend time together as a new family.

part of the newborn's life, providing a kind of bridge from the time in the womb to post-birth experience and laying the groundwork for a basic sense of security in later life. Yet studies have also shown that children whose fathers are involved in their lives from birth fare better cognitively, academically, and socially as they grow. Clearly, a child's healthiest growth springs from a secure attachment to *both* parents.

Did You Know . . .

FACTS ABOUT BREASTFEEDING

- Breastfeeding babies tend to be healthier than formula-fed babies—and you won't have to deal with bottles, expensive cans of formula, or other equipment. You will save money that you would have spent to purchase formula.

- Breastfeeding has been shown to reduce the risk of breast, ovarian, and endometrial cancer in a mother's later life and may reduce the risk of osteoporosis.
- Breastfeeding women use the weight (fat stores) they accumulated during pregnancy to produce breast milk.
- Women who breastfeed for more than twelve months during their lifetime tend to have lower risk of high blood pressure, high cholesterol, heart disease, and diabetes.
- A mother's perception of her partner's attitude toward breastfeeding is one of the greatest factors influencing her decision to breastfeed.
- Exclusive breastfeeding, with no supplemental formula or solid feedings, delays the mother's ovulation and works as a natural form of birth control for the first six months after childbirth, if the mother has not resumed her menstrual cycles and if her baby is continuing to breastfeed fully both day and through the night.
- A breastfeeding mother whose partner supports her by taking care of household responsibilities is likely to be more successful and keep breastfeeding longer, enjoy family life more, and have more energy left over for her adult relationships.
- Babies' brain development depends on frequent verbal, physical, and emotional interaction with a familiar, loving caregiver. Babies need to be sung to, rocked, and played with as much as they need time breastfeeding. The baby needs these things and they will not spoil her.
- Eye contact between parent and infant is important for infant development. Mother and baby frequently make eye contact during breastfeeding. The non-breastfeeding partner can maintain eye contact while changing her diaper, giving her a bath, and playing with her.

- Growing children benefit from experiencing the different but complementary parenting styles of two different adults.
- The American Academy of Pediatrics recommends breastfeeding as the sole source of nutrition for infants for about the first six months, breastfeeding in combination with solid foods for the next six months, and continued breastfeeding thereafter for as long as mutually desired by mother and baby.

HOW CAN I HELP? (AND WHAT'S IN IT FOR ME?)

It is easy to say that the significant other is important in the lives of the newborn and partner, but it can be hard at times to see *how* to participate—especially during the early months. It may help to keep in mind that little things mean a great deal at this time: a word of encouragement for your partner as she adjusts to her new routine, an offer to help with the housework or care for the baby while she takes a nap, or a confident defense when a friend or relative questions her decision to breastfeed on demand. These small acts let your partner know that you firmly support her decision to breastfeed and that you'll continue to support her. Many studies have shown the support of a loving partner is the most important deciding factor in whether or not a woman chooses to initiate and continue breastfeeding. After all, you are the baby's other parent and perhaps your partner's closest friend. By seconding the decision to give your child the best possible nourishment, your actions can have a decisive and immediate impact on your baby's life.

One of the first steps you can take as the partner of a breastfeeding mother is to educate yourself regarding breastfeeding's many benefits. You are already doing that by reading this chapter (and, hopefully, the rest of this book). You might also ask your baby's pediatrician to discuss the advantages of breast milk over formula and give you an idea what to expect in practical terms during your baby's first few months of life. If at all possible, attend breastfeeding classes with your partner. By understanding how breastfeeding is accomplished, you can better help your partner after the birth as she learns such techniques as positioning your baby for proper latch-on. Remember that many people still are not aware of the tremendous benefits of breastfeeding and have not been part of a breastfeeding relationship.

Immediately after birth you can support your partner's decision to begin breastfeeding by helping to make her comfortable in the delivery room. While in the hospital, you can take turns holding, rocking, and changing diapers so she can sleep between feedings. Also, you can support your mutual decision that the baby is not to receive a pacifier, a bottle, or supplemental formula without a clear medical reason. If your baby is unable to breastfeed due to

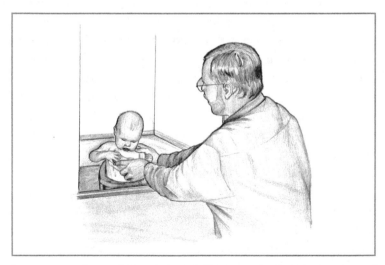

Partners can take an active role in their baby's care by bathing, changing, and burping the baby.

an illness, you can ask to have a breast pump for your partner and help her get it ready for use.

Once you are all home from the hospital and family life has begun, your role as the partner of a breastfeeding mother will take on a new importance. As your baby's mother concentrates on establishing her breastfeeding routine, you can focus on keeping the household running efficiently and acting as a buffer for possible distractions to successful breastfeeding. If possible, take some time off work to prepare meals, keep up with the laundry, keep older children entertained, and otherwise allow mother and new baby to concentrate on learning to breastfeed and getting the rest they need.

Offer your partner food and drink while she's nursing, bring her pillows if she needs them to position the baby, and provide her with a book, telephone, diapers, or whatever else she likes to have near at hand. If you see that she's having trouble nursing—if she experiences discomfort with breastfeeding or she worries that the baby's not getting enough milk—use your own observations and insights to help her make adjustments in the feeding technique. If you see that she's still struggling but is reluctant to ask for help, assist her to seek outside professional help, and tell her that you are there to assist in any way possible. She will appreciate your concern and steadfast support.

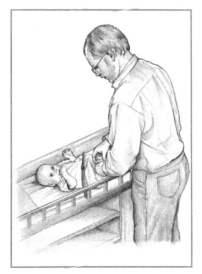

As you and your partner become more familiar with the routines of parenting, you can help with diaper changes, baths, and playtimes so your partner can sleep between feedings and perhaps enjoy a little time to herself. These interactions with

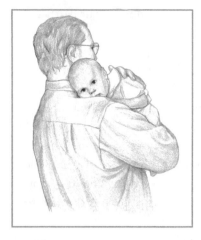

your newborn are excellent opportunities for you to create your own unique relationship with him. In the beginning, your baby will have less "awake time," but as the baby gets older, you will find that the baby has more time to play.

After feeding, a content baby is usually happy to snuggle up against your chest for a nap or may be ready to play. Make the most of these moments—smiling and talking with your baby as you change his diaper, playfully splashing him in the bathtub if he enjoys getting splashed, holding and rocking him when he cries, and making up fun little games that he plays only with you. Babies also love to be part of such "grown-up" activities as taking a walk outside and "reading" books and magazines. As your child regularly experiences these times with you, he will understand that you are your own special parent and not just a substitute for Mommy.

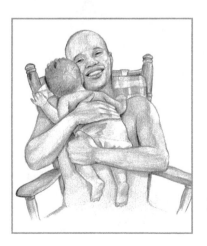

Babies love to snuggle after a feeding, a great opportunity for fathers to bond with their babies.

Pitching In

TIPS FROM EXPERIENCED PARTNERS

- **It's the little things.** A word of encouragement or an offer to hold the baby can mean a lot to the mother and keep your home life more upbeat. Keep your eyes open for ways to convey these messages, such as bringing flowers home after work, telling your partner she looks beautiful, letting her know you appreciate her breastfeeding your child, and getting up first in the morning to take care of household chores so she can sleep.

- **Focus on the baby.** Once the baby is born, your baby's mother may be preoccupied with learning new skills, relatives may offer conflicting advice, and your own work-and-parenting routine may feel overwhelming at times. It can be tempting to step back and let your partner handle new parenthood—but she will need your help in establishing breastfeeding. Think about your baby's needs and figure out how you can meet them most effectively.

- **Remember, this time won't last.** At first, chances are you'll both feel tired or frustrated now and then. Talk ahead of time about what to do when you're tempted to snap at each other. A private joke, a kiss, or an offer to talk things through may defuse the situation. Keep in mind that what you are doing is important and you won't be new parents for long. Appreciate this amazing, unique period while it lasts.

- **Get to know your child.** This is your baby too. Introduce him to your world, observe his responses, and begin enjoying your unique relationship.

∽   COMBINING WORK AND FAMILY LIFE

Work schedules pose additional challenges to both parents of a breastfeeding child. If you work outside the home during the early months of parenthood, you will need to monitor your energy supply as carefully as your partner does. Try not to extend your work hours, take on extra projects, or travel much during this period if possible. If you find that you or your partner are feeling seriously sleep-deprived, discuss ways to reallocate parenting time so you both can have the time for sleep and relaxation that you need.

If and when your child's mother begins working outside the home, she will need the same consideration from you. Adjusting to her new responsibilities can be daunting at first as she meets such challenges as learning how to use a breast pump, storing breast milk for future use, arranging for child care, and expressing milk on the job. You may be able to make this process easier in one of many ways—such as helping locate a suitable caregiver, packing the baby's bag before work each morning, cleaning or preparing the breast pump at night for the next day's use, and making sure

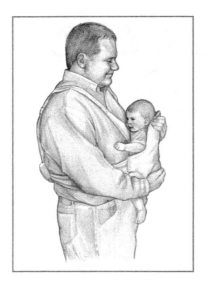

Your partner can help you by playing with or carrying the baby, assisting in finding a caregiver, and washing and preparing breast pumps for use.

mother and baby enjoy an undisturbed "reunion feeding" at the end of each workday. You may also consider taking your child, when feasible, to the mother's workplace for a midday feeding. Keep in mind, too, that your partner may be more tired than usual as she learns to combine motherhood with a job. Make allowances for her limited reserves and work to keep the lines of communication open.

Of course, you can get tired and just plain discouraged, too, and at these times it helps to have a few people in mind who know how to help you relax and let off steam. Ideally, you will enjoy the support of close friends who also participated a great deal in raising their babies. Such experienced parents can offer solutions for problems, sympathy when things get tough, and suggestions on dealing with the unsought advice and criticism that some new parents receive. If you don't know any parents who have played an active role in the lives of their children, contact your local La Leche League (see Chapter 3) for information on couples meetings. Finally, don't forget your friends or associates at work, who can empathize with many aspects of parenting life and offer insights about situations that concern you. Whomever you choose to talk to, make sure you do take the time to talk. Becoming a parent is an enormous transition for every couple. Sharing both the highs and the lows with an empathetic friend will enhance and deepen your experience.

BREASTFEEDING AND SEXUALITY

I'd heard all the jokes about what a new baby does to your sex life, a father wrote, *but when it happened to us, I felt like our marriage had been hit with a truck. All of a sudden, my wife didn't want to be touched anymore—ever! That was a hard part of adjusting to parenthood, but now we're back the way we were. Actually, I'd say our relationship is even more satisfying now than it was before our daughter was born.*

It really shouldn't be surprising that the experience of childbirth, a significant amount of sleep deprivation, and a radically new family structure can create some very strong shock waves in a couple's relationship. Many parents are startled by the swings in their feelings about each other and their desire for sexual contact. Complicating things more is the fact that each parent's experiences differ in such important ways at first—with mothers in almost constant physical contact with their babies while partners look on, desiring more closeness. At the end of the day, a new mother may have had so much "touching" that sex is the last thing on her mind, while the non-breastfeeding partner may feel especially in need of some physical sign of her affection.

This is not always the case, of course. Some breastfeeding mothers (and their partners) experience less sexual desire during certain phases of parenthood, while others experience more. If you and your partner find that the intimacy of the breastfeeding period enhances your sexual life, or if you feel freed by the natural birth control benefits of exclusive breastfeeding during the first six months, take full advantage of it. If, on the other hand, your desires conflict, try to remember that this stage will pass, and focus on keeping the lines of communication open in the meantime. Remember that intimacy is not equated with having sexual intercourse; rather, it's important that you and your partner feel a closeness and bond with each other. Kisses, an occasional nuzzle, or a back rub may convey these feelings better than more intense physical contact. Sincere compliments can mean a lot to a new mother, who may feel less "put together" than she's used to and may feel a little self-conscious about her postpartum shape.

While couples may feel that their sexual life has changed with the birth of the baby, studies have shown that most couples resume intercourse at about seven weeks postpartum, though breastfeeding couples' sexual activity tends to resume more gradually than that of bottle-feeding couples throughout the first year. By taking into account this typical pattern of sexual activity and understanding that it's a normal part of the transition from pregnancy to life as a family, you may be able to relax enough during this temporary

Pillow Talk

HOW DO YOU FEEL ABOUT BREASTFEEDING?

In a recent study, pregnant women were asked to predict what their partners' attitudes toward breastfeeding would be. Surprisingly, their responses were highly inaccurate (hardly better than random guessing). Most believed that their partners were far more negative about breastfeeding than they actually were. For this reason, it's important to share your feelings about breastfeeding and new parenthood with your partner whenever possible. Such conversations can help preserve the intimacy of your relationship during the physically challenging early months, while also supporting your partner in her breastfeeding efforts at a time when every encouraging word helps. If you love the sight of her breastfeeding your baby, tell her how it makes you feel. If you consider her nursing mother's figure just as sexy, let her know Share with her your pride in her commitment to breastfeeding as she breastfeeds in public and makes herself available to satisfy your child's hunger at all times. Such words of support and affirmation can act as a highly effective aphrodisiac for many new mothers (if not now, then later) and may improve your relationship even as they ensure your child's continued good health.

glitch in your sex life to enjoy the wonderful changes that are happening in your family.

I'LL GET HIM, YOU SLEEP: CREATING A PARENTING TEAM

As the non-breastfeeding partner, you should work with your child's mother to create a routine that works best for your family's lifestyle. For starters, have an honest discussion about how you plan to divide parenting duties. Who will get him when he cries before you're heading to bed? Who will handle the mornings? When should your baby take a bottle from you? Then plan your schedules accordingly. If you know that you'll be getting your baby when he awakens at 6:00 a.m., you'll feel less guilty about letting Mom retrieve him at 3:00 a.m. for a middle-of-the-night nursing. You may find you actually enjoy taking charge of your baby and being his primary caregiver while you let his mother sleep. And at night after work, you may offer to take your baby while your child's mother catches a quick nap or enjoys a shower. Relieving her stress will mean she has more energy for you.

By stepping up and assuming your responsibilities for your baby, you'll begin to view yourself as a valuable part of the parenting team. As an added bonus, you and your baby will begin to forge a special bond. The additional responsibilities will also help you appreciate the energy it takes for your child's mother to be a breastfeeding mom. And remember, in the end, it's your baby who will benefit most from having the time and affection of both parents.

Q & A

Can I Do Something?

Q: *My partner believes strongly in breastfeeding on demand, but my parents think she's spoiling our three-week-old by nursing her every hour or even more frequently. They tell me that at this rate our child will never learn responsibility and self-control and that she'll grow up expecting to boss us around. Who's right—my partner or my parents? And how do I keep them all happy?*

A: Your parents' response to breastfeeding on demand is a quite common belief but inappropriate, as was discussed in Chapter 6. A three-week-old baby is incapable of being spoiled and can only benefit from learning that her needs will consistently be met. You may not be able to change your parents' view, but it is important to express to them that you agree with the mother's decision to breastfeed whenever her child wishes. Your partner will appreciate your support and the fact that you and she are united in your decisions. By backing her up, you are creating a powerful parenting team that will serve the family well in the years to come. Chances are that eventually your parents will see that both of you made the right decision.

Q: *Our baby boy, Henry, is eight weeks old and has not yet slept through an entire night. My partner is exhausted, so lately I've been trying to give her a break by getting up to play with Henry for a while before she breastfeeds. Unfortunately, Henry just keeps crying the entire time, louder and louder, until his mother gets up and takes him. Is there some way I can make him happy so my partner can sleep?*

A: Your baby's cries are his way of telling you that he's hungry and needs to be fed. By responding to his needs, you increase his trust and attachment to you, thus laying the groundwork for healthy growth throughout his childhood. Tired as your partner might be, it's important for her to nurse your baby when he communicates his need. You can make night feedings easier by carrying the baby to her, letting her nurse while still in bed and half asleep, and then changing his diaper and helping him get back to sleep. Consider keeping your baby close by in a cradle or crib next to the bed so she doesn't have to get up to get him. Many couples assign the "day shift" to one parent and the "night shift" to the other—so that, for example, the breastfeeding mom tends to the baby at night, but after the first morning feeding, the partner gets up with him and takes care of his needs as much as possible during the day between feedings. Soon feedings will decrease in frequency and your son will sleep for longer intervals. Meanwhile, your partner and child will be grateful for your help.

Q: *My wife and I separated during her pregnancy and she has custody of the baby. I would like to set up a visitation schedule with my baby. Is this possible with a breastfeeding infant?*

A: You are off to an excellent start as a parent by recognizing your child's need to breastfeed as a top priority at this time. Ideally, you will be able to work with the baby's mother to create a visitation schedule that allows for this need, rather than relying on a court-mandated arrangement that might be less favorable. The best visitation schedule starts with the length and frequency of separations from the mother that your baby already experiences, and gradually lengthens as time passes. If the mother doesn't work outside the home and breastfeeds on demand, you will need to begin with frequent, brief visits (perhaps visiting the child for an hour before work, during lunch, or after work on appointed days, preferably in the mother's home). If he is accustomed to longer separations with a caregiver, you can take the caregiver's place for the same length of time. As you increase the number and length of your visits with your child, discuss with his mother the possibility of using a bottle to feed him breast milk she has expressed with a pump or by hand—and keep in mind that you will be able to feed him other foods after he is six months old. Once you have reached this stage and feedings are spaced apart more, it becomes easier for you to go out with your child for a brief time. Eventually he will be able to happily stay overnight and on weekends with you.

CHAPTER 12

Weaning Your Baby

Your sister weaned her daughter at eight months; your best friend stopped when her son was two. Now that your daughter is a year old, you're noticing that she's starting to lose interest in nursing. Knowing exactly when to wean your baby isn't always easy, but it's an inevitable event for any nursing mother. The key is doing it gradually and making sure that both you and your baby are ready for this transition.

IS THIS GOODBYE?

The decision to stop breastfeeding is a personal choice, and many mothers are surprised that their own goals and desires in this area differ markedly from those of other mothers and even from those of their children. Chances are both of you have enjoyed the closeness that comes with breastfeeding. In fact, you may want to continue nursing your child through toddlerhood. But your child's active temperament may cause him to be too impatient to continue to nurse. On the other hand, your child may want to continue nursing long past his first year, particularly before bedtime and when he's in need of comfort. But you may feel the need to move on to new activities. Whenever and for whatever reason you decide that the time has come (or, as is sometimes the case, suddenly realize that feedings have tapered off almost of their own accord), look at this change as another positive step in your life together and a window into the fascinating new ways your child is growing.

IS THIS THE RIGHT TIME? WHEN TO WEAN

Planning ahead when to stop breastfeeding—or trying to decide what the best age for weaning might be—can be a particularly difficult exercise for parents in this country. Few if any cultural conventions tell us precisely when it is time to completely wean from the breast, yet concerned relatives and friends often seem to have strong opinions about what's best for the child and mother. The American Academy of Pediatrics recommends continued breastfeeding beyond the first birthday as long as mutually desired by mother and child. However, mothers in the United States have tended to wean much earlier than in most other countries. At the end of 2006, 21 percent of U.S. mothers breastfed for a year. For black mothers this rate was only 12 percent, and for mothers younger than twenty years it was 8 percent. In addition, weaning is more often initiated by the mother in this country, whereas in most other cultures children begin the process when they feel ready. Worldwide, the average age for weaning is between two and four, and in some societies breastfeeding continues up to age six or seven. Today, though, later weaning is steadily gaining wider acceptance in the general population.

Scientific research on the benefits of long-term breastfeeding for the health and well-being of child and mother is growing. Researchers have found that the composition of the mother's milk continues to change during her baby's second year of life, and it continues to provide important nutritional benefits and to bolster the toddler's immune system. Studies have also demonstrated evidence of a "dose effect" for breastfeeding—meaning that the longer breastfeeding continues and the more breast milk a child consumes, the better the health for child and mother. Further research has shown that the longer children are breastfed in their first

An Experience of a Lifetime

COMMON FEELINGS ABOUT WEANING

Breastfeeding mothers' feelings about ending this period of their lives are as varied and intense as any other basic parenting experience. You may be surprised at how powerful and even turbulent your emotional response is to the idea of weaning your baby—whether you can hardly imagine no longer nursing or long for greater freedom. Some mothers may feel sad about giving up the closeness that comes from breastfeeding. Others may feel ambivalence between desire for greater independence from their babies and a longing for continued closeness.

Whatever your feelings about this major transition (and you may well experience all of them at one time or another), understand that such emotional responses are quite common and natural. By cuddling and interacting with your baby even more during the weaning process, you will start to stabilize your own emotions and adjust to this new stage in your life as a mother. Talk with friends who have experienced weaning with their own children, or write down your own experiences to share with your child when she's grown. Finally, remember that weaning is a natural step in helping your child grow up. You will both make it through this transition and thrive as you find new ways to remain close.

year of life, the better they perform in tests of cognitive skills and academic achievement. This especially holds true for children who are breastfed for more than eight months. Certain health benefits of breastfeeding rely on longer durations of feeding, such as protection from childhood cancers such as leukemia and lymphoma. Additional cancer protection occurs with prolonged breastfeeding for the mother, with a much lower likelihood of breast cancer after total lifetime breastfeeding for two years. For these and many other reasons, the World Health Organization recommends exclusive breastfeeding for six months and urges mothers to continue breastfeeding at least until their child is two years old.

The simplest, most natural time to wean is when your child initiates the process. Weaning begins naturally at six months, when iron-fortified solid foods are introduced. Even after introduction of complementary foods, infants take similar volumes of human milk. Other fluids, however, will limit your baby's desire to take as much human milk and may hasten the weaning process. Some infants begin to turn gradually away from breastfeeding and toward other forms of nutrition and comfort at around one year of age, when they have begun to enjoy a wide variety of solid foods and have learned to drink from a cup. Others wean themselves during the toddler years as they become more physically active and less willing to sit still to nurse. Gradually tapering off the number of nursing sessions—by eliminating a feeding every two or three days—at this time can ensure that the weaning process will proceed quite smoothly, as your child becomes so busy with new experiences that she forgets it's time to nurse.

You may, however, decide to initiate weaning at an earlier time for reasons of your own. These may include the need to be away

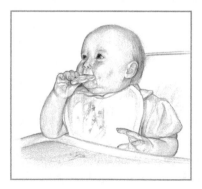

Older babies enjoy self-feeding as they demonstrate new independence and experience new tastes and textures.

from home for longer periods, a new pregnancy, job constraints, or even an increasing lack of desire to breastfeed. (It is important to remember, though, that you *can* continue to breastfeed even if you have become pregnant or return to work, perhaps reducing the frequency of breastfeeding and incorporating some use of infant formula.) Starting the weaning process yourself will not be as easy as following your child's lead, but with care and sensitivity it can certainly be accomplished. Meanwhile, it's important to focus on your child's needs and your own. Be selective in following the inevitable advice and judgment of others outside the mother-child relationship, resist comparing your situation to that of any other family, and maybe even rethink any advance deadlines you set for yourself when you were pregnant or your child was a newborn. Keep in mind that you have provided the best start for your baby by breastfeeding, no matter how early or late you decide to stop. Some breastfeeding is better than none. No one but you can decide what is best for you and your infant.

To Wean or Not to Wean

WHEN PARENTS DISAGREE

Many mothers—particularly those breastfeeding their first babies—are surprised at how much family tradition, cultural background, and the opinions of others come into play as they consider the optimal time for weaning. As fathers in this country become more involved in the parenting process in general, they are also likely to have opinions—sometimes quite strong ones— about when breastfeeding is appropriate and at what age it is not. If your child's father comes from a family whose traditions favor breastfeeding into toddlerhood, he may disapprove of your desire to stop breastfeeding at, say, your child's first birthday. If his own mother did not breastfeed or clearly disapproves of your continuing to nurse, he may pressure you to wean sooner than you or your baby would like.

When facing such a situation, it is necessary to recognize the father's desire to "do the right thing" for you and your child and to appreciate the powerful forces that affect his opinion. If you feel that his decisions on the matter spring more from the sense that "that's the way it has always been done" rather than from conclusions based on scientific evidence and expert advice, suggest that he read this book and ask your pediatrician or La Leche League volunteer (see Chapter 3) to refer you to a parenting group or fathers' club that addresses this issue in the context of general child development. Finally, listen carefully to the reasons he gives for his opinions. The final decision of when to wean should remain with you and your child, but by focusing on Dad's issues and finding other ways to satisfy his goals (allowing more time for him and his baby between nursing sessions, for instance), you can turn this conflict into an opportunity for growth and greater understanding for the entire family. If conflict persists, consult your pediatrician or family physician for additional help.

A GRADUAL PARTING: HOW TO WEAN

As indicated previously, weaning is a natural process, and it's best for you and your child if it happens in a natural way. The key word in this context is *gradual*—a gradual move toward other forms of nutrition and closeness, with the number and length of breastfeeding sessions tapering off over weeks or even months. In this way, you and your child will have time to find other ways to maintain closeness, express and accept tenderness or comfort, and ensure

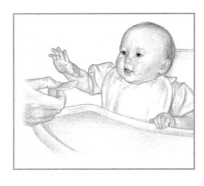

Exposing a child to new foods during a regular breastfeeding time may help him wean.

proper nutritional intake before you completely stop nursing. You will also avoid the conflicts and resistance that tend to spring from more abrupt weaning and even minimize your own physical difficulties such as breast engorgement.

One of the most effective ways to begin a gradual weaning process with a child age one or older is simply not to offer a feeding and wait to see if he requests it. The easiest first session to skip

A Healthy Substitute

INSTEAD OF HUMAN MILK . . .

Your child's age is important in determining what kinds of nourishment to offer in place of human milk during the weaning process. Babies under age one should receive iron-fortified formula, not whole cow's milk. In general, children ages one to two can have whole milk. Reduced-fat milk, either low-fat or skim, is appropriate for children age two and older who are drinking cow's milk. Recent evidence suggests, however, that if weight is a problem, a toddler between one and two years may be fed low-fat cow's milk.

in this way is usually the midday breastfeeding, when your child may already have had access to a lunch of solid food and such liquids as cow's milk or fruit juice. Your child may well become so interested in another activity after lunch that he forgets about nursing and never requests a midday feeding again. If your child does signal a desire to nurse, however, be sure to satisfy his desire. In weaning, as in all developmental processes, it's best to follow your child's lead. In any case, refusing to breastfeed will only increase his desire and focus his attention on the activity. Distracting him with new foods or different kinds of interaction during his usual breastfeeding time is a more positive and effective way to help him wean.

Once your child has grown accustomed to missing the midday nursing session, take a look at skipping a second feeding in the same manner. Again, redirecting his attention to new activities, other food options, and sources of emotional reassurance (such as a favorite blanket or stuffed animal) will help him make the transition more easily. If he decides that he still wants to nurse, offer the breast, thus reassuring him that you are still there for him as he continues to explore his surroundings. If he clings to one or two favorite feeding times—usually the last one before bedtime and the first one in the morning—consider continuing these sessions for as long as he wants to nurse. Such quiet times rarely interfere with even the busiest family's schedule and are a wonderful way to maintain that special closeness with your child.

Some mothers find that it is not so much the transition to other activities that challenges young children in the midst of the weaning process but the difficulty of adapting to new feeding methods such as a bottle or a cup. This is particularly true of infants and younger toddlers. In Chapter 9, methods to help your baby make the transition from breastfeeding to drinking expressed milk from a cup or bottle were presented. The same methods can be used to move your child toward formula (if he is less than one year old) or milk (age one and older) during weaning. Keep in

Not Quite Yet . . .

WHEN NOT TO WEAN

In most cases, the decision to wean can be based on a mother's and child's inner needs and practical considerations relating to the family. However, it's best to put off weaning in some situations until a time when conditions are better. Such situations include:

- **Food allergies.** If you or your child's father have experienced food allergies, talk with your child's pediatrician or other health professional about the benefits of delaying weaning until at least after your child's first birthday. As pointed out in Chapter 7, avoiding cow's milk or cow's-milk-based products may be helpful.
- **Illness.** If your child has a cold, is teething, has recently been hospitalized, or is otherwise not in tip-top shape, put off initiating the weaning process until he feels better. You might also want to delay your first attempts if you feel under the weather. It's always best to meet any transition period when you and your child are at your physical and emotional best.
- **Changes at home.** If you are pregnant or have recently had a new baby, this may not be the best time to wean, unless led by your child. On the other hand, your needs and the needs of a newborn may take priority. Always breastfeed the newborn first, but try to be sensitive to the needs of everyone involved. Likewise, a move to a new home, a marital disruption, a new child care situation, your return to work, and other potentially stressful situations are not the best times to initiate another major change. Ideally, you will begin weaning when it's not overly stressful for you or your child.

mind, though, that if you choose to wean your child to a bottle, you will have to wean to a cup later on. For best dental hygiene and to prevent tooth decay, babies older than nine months of age should be transitioned to a cup rather than a bottle.

You can use the same gradual method of substitution when introducing a younger baby to a bottle or cup as you would with an older child. If you decide to use a bottle, introduce it gradually over several days. Use it with one feeding—probably the midday session—and work your way up to more. It helps if your baby is not extremely hungry, because then he may be more patient when trying out the cup or bottle. Pay attention to your baby's responses. Some breastfed babies accept a bottle more easily if someone other than the mother offers it. (But some prefer taking a bottle while in their mother's arms.) If you or another adult have tried for several days to get your baby to accept a bottle and he has continued to refuse, try changing to a different kind of nipple for a few days or switch to a cup. If your baby uses a pacifier, he may prefer a similar nipple for feedings. Babies can be particular about the type of nipple they use, but once they are introduced to one they like, they may adjust easily. Meanwhile, during this learning process, don't force your baby to take a bottle. The process of bottle-feeding is quite different from breastfeeding, and his adjustment may well take time. Excess pressure to take a bottle may cause him to refuse the bottle (see Chapter 9).

After bottle-feedings have started, some babies get frustrated when nursing, because the milk doesn't flow as fast from the breast as from the bottle. If this is the case with your child, try offering him the breast before he gets too hungry and is too impatient to adapt to its naturally slower flow. Help your milk flow faster by massaging the breast as you nurse. (Pumping for one or two minutes before starting to breastfeed can start your milk flowing faster too.) A bottle with a slow-flowing nipple may also help diminish the difference between the bottle-feeding and breastfeeding experiences.

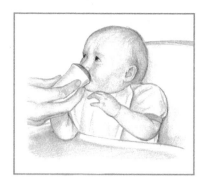

Some breastfed babies transition more readily to drinking from a cup than a bottle.

Many mothers, particularly those whose babies are older, prefer to wean directly to a cup—thus eliminating the need to wean their child from the bottle later on. (A bottle can become a beloved security object for a child age one or older, and persuading him to give it up can turn into quite a challenge.) To introduce your baby to a cup, start with a small plastic one or, even better, a trainer cup with a snap-on lid to prevent spills and two handles for your baby to grasp. Don't be surprised if he treats the cup as a toy at first. He will probably throw it nearly as often as he drinks from it. This is perfectly normal baby or toddler behavior and part of the process of familiarizing himself with this new tool.

It is often the case when raising children that our best-laid parenting plans are disrupted by the realities of our particular children's personalities, needs, and situations. Even when you have made the time and taken care to proceed with weaning in a leisurely manner, your child may elect to cut down nursing quite abruptly or stop breastfeeding altogether. His desire to make this transition today instead of tomorrow is in no way a rejection of you but a sign of his independence. Likewise, if your child continues to need to nurse for longer than you had planned, do not interpret this as a sign that he is immature, lacks self-confidence, or is overly dependent on you. Instead, you can be reassured that your child still values breastfeeding and receives security and comfort from cuddling during nursing.

Slow Down!

PHYSICAL CHANGES DURING WEANING

When weaning is accomplished gradually, mothers of older babies and toddlers sometimes hardly notice at first that their milk has diminished and that other changes are taking place. One of the most important physical changes to note as your child moves from exclusive breastfeeding toward partial breastfeeding with the addition of formula, cow's milk, or solids is the gradual return of your hormones to their pre-pregnancy state. This is associated with the normal cycling of your estrogen and progesterone levels, with release of eggs, and the possibility of becoming pregnant. This possibility increases naturally after the baby reaches six months. Should you not want to become pregnant again right away, discuss alternative methods of birth control with your gynecologist and your partner (refer to Chapter 6 for a discussion of these methods), and be sure to begin using some type of birth control immediately.

Changes in your breasts will take place more gradually, even in cases when the weaning process itself moves at a brisk pace. You may continue to produce some milk for months after your child has stopped nursing, particularly if your nipples continue to be stimulated or you otherwise check to see whether milk is still present. It will also probably take several months for your breasts to return to their pre-pregnancy size. After weaning, some women find that their breasts are slightly different in size or firmness than before their pregnancy. You should continue to perform monthly breast self-examinations throughout breastfeeding, including the weaning period, and bring any concerns about lumps or firmness to your doctor's attention.

Breast pain caused by engorgement should not be a problem

if you proceed with weaning gradually. Your breasts will simply slow down milk production as demand decreases until little is produced and finally none. If your child has elected to stop nursing more abruptly, however, you may experience some discomfort. If this is the case, express just enough milk to keep your breasts from feeling so full. Keep in mind that expressing more than a small amount of milk will spur greater milk production and increase discomfort even more. (Persistent, unrelieved engorgement may increase your risk of developing mastitis, an infection and/or inflammation of the breast.) Meanwhile, try to encourage your child to wean more gradually, if possible. You don't want to force him to breastfeed if he's not interested, of course, but slowing down the weaning pace a bit could make the process more comfortable for you. This process may also signal that your little one is ready to move on to a new stage in your relationship.

IF YOUR CHILD RESISTS

Some children strongly object to their mother's efforts to move from breast to bottle or cup, no matter how sensitively and gradually the process is approached. This resistance can become frustrating if you want or need to wean by a specific time (for example, if you need to start back to work or school and have decided not to express your milk during your separation). Unfortunately, the more anxious you become about completing the weaning process, the more difficult it may become as your baby picks up on your feelings of impatience.

The best approach is to take a deep breath, remember that this too shall pass, and review the previous section for additional ad-

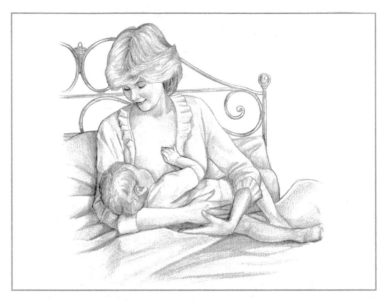

Your toddler may turn to nursing for comfort and reassurance and will still receive nutritional and immunologic benefits.

vice. Consider shortening your nursing sessions as a prelude to dropping them altogether. At the times of day when your child is used to nursing, stay away from your usual nursing locations, involve her in an interesting activity, and avoid such strong nursing cues as pulling her onto your lap, uncovering your breasts in front of her, or even sitting down. Don't forget to offer her even more than the usual amount of affection, hugs, and kisses, though. The emotional component of breastfeeding is powerful for the older baby and toddler and is best replaced with other forms of physical contact and expressions of your love.

If your baby still resists, consider whether you might continue breastfeeding—just less often—while offering a cup, bottle, or other foods at other times. By partially weaning (for example, initially keeping the early-morning and before-bed feedings, and then gradually dropping the early-morning session), you eliminate a source of conflict between your child and yourself that may turn out to be unnecessary. You also send your child the message that you are paying attention to her feelings and responding to them. Eventually you can agree with your older child on an endpoint for nursing. In the meantime, your willingness to recognize her needs and provide for them sets an excellent pattern in your relationship for the years to come.

PLAY WITH ME! A NEW RELATIONSHIP WITH YOUR CHILD

No doubt the end of your breastfeeding experience marks a milestone in your relationship with your child. And while you may feel some sadness at first and even envy toward other moms who are still nursing, you'll soon notice that your child will do just fine without breastfeeding—and that you'll be just fine too. You and your child will certainly find new and exciting ways to enjoy your relationship. Rest assured that if you plan to have children in the future, you'll certainly have the opportunity to share that same special breastfeeding relationship with them as well.

For now, you can congratulate yourself on a job well done as you complete this stage of your breastfeeding relationship with your child. Being a nursing mother takes a tremendous amount of knowledge, effort, and time, but it is also one of the most rewarding experiences you can have. As you watch your baby grow into a healthy, confident, secure child, you will see those first lessons in love and commitment take root and enhance her ability to make friends and communicate with others. Someday, when she is a parent to her own newborn, perhaps she will experience the same special bond in breastfeeding that you found in feeding and nurturing her.

Q&A

Does She Still Need Me?

Q: *I have just learned that I must have surgery a week from now. I'm afraid that breastfeeding will be too difficult during my recovery, and I'm thinking about weaning over the next seven days. Can I wean my baby in such a short time?*

A: As noted in Chapter 5, few types of surgery require a woman to stop breastfeeding entirely. In cases that require a temporary interruption in breastfeeding, consider expressing your milk before the surgery and freezing it for your baby's use until you can resume nursing. Abrupt weaning should be attempted only when no alternative presents itself. If you must end breastfeeding in a brief time, try following the steps laid out in the previous sections of this chapter, but speed them up somewhat. Apply cabbage leaves to your breasts to ease your discomfort (see pages 150–151). Your child may resist the accelerated pace, but you will at least have introduced her to alternative feeding possibilities before you wean completely. Be sure to make time for a great deal of cuddling, playing, and other non-nursing-related contact to cushion any feelings of confusion your child may experience. Meanwhile, keep in mind your own need to adjust to this sudden change by easing breast engorgement (see above) and making allowances for hormonal and emotional fluctuations.

Q: *My toddler seems to get most of his calories from solid foods and cow's milk and wants to breastfeed only when he's upset or tired. Is it healthy to continue breastfeeding if nursing has turned into a comfort ritual more than anything else?*

A: Your toddler may turn to nursing for comfort and reassurance, but he is certainly still benefiting from the nutritional and immuno-

logic benefits. In any case, emotional support is a perfectly legitimate aspect of breastfeeding. Seeking out a reassuring nursing session when he's upset and bouncing back as soon as he finishes
builds your child's confidence and feelings of security and well-
being. Certainly there is no evidence that extended breastfeeding
makes a child more dependent or harms him in any way. On the
contrary, many parents proudly tell how independent, healthy, and
exceptionally bright their long-term breastfed children become. As
long as you are comfortable breastfeeding your toddler, there is no
reason to stop.

Q: *My three-year-old is nearly weaned but still has a hard time falling
asleep without nursing. Is it okay to nurse her to sleep, or should I insist
that she learn to fall asleep on her own?*
A: Falling asleep at the breast is a profoundly satisfying experience
for a young child—one she has probably enjoyed from her earliest
days. While it is true that children need to explore different ways to
let go of wakefulness at the end of the day, a nursing session just before bedtime can help your daughter relax enough to focus on this
skill and succeed at it. Since any kind of milk or juice can promote
tooth decay when in contact with your baby's teeth for long periods, try offering your child the breast just before brushing her teeth
and then ease her toward sleep with a bedtime story and a kiss
good-night.

Breastfeeding Resources

Professional Organizations and Website Directory

American Academy of Pediatrics
141 Northwest Point Boulevard
Elk Grove Village, IL 60007
847-434-4000
www.HealthyChildren.org
The American Academy of Pediatrics is an organization of sixty thousand pediatricians dedicated to the health, safety, and well-being of infants, children, adolescents, and young adults. Its website for parents, HealthyChildren.org, offers trustworthy, up-to-the-minute health care information and guidance for parents and caregivers along with interactive tools and personalized content. You can also get answers to specific questions by clicking on "Ask a Pediatrician."

Academy of Breastfeeding Medicine
140 Huguenot Street, 3rd Floor
New Rochelle, NY 10801
(800) 990-4ABM
(914) 740-2115
www.bfmed.org
The Academy of Breastfeeding Medicine is an international organization of physicians with expertise or interest in breastfeeding promotion, education, support, and research.

American Dietetic Association
120 South Riverside Plaza, Suite 2000
Chicago, IL 60606-6995
(800) 877-1600
(312) 899-0040
www.eatright.org
The American Dietetic Association is the world's largest organization of food and nutrition professionals. ADA is committed to improving the nation's health and advancing the profession of dietetics through research, education, and advocacy.

Baby-Friendly USA, Inc.
327 Quaker Meeting House Road
East Sandwich, MA 02537
(508) 888-8092
www.babyfriendlyusa.org
The Baby-Friendly Hospital Initiative is an international program of the World Health Organization (WHO) and the United Nations Children's Fund (UNICEF). Based on the WHO/UNICEF Ten Steps to Successful Breastfeeding, the initiative recognizes hospitals and birth centers that have taken steps to provide an optimal environment for the promotion, protection, and support of breastfeeding. Baby-Friendly USA is the organization that oversees implementation of the Baby-Friendly Hospital Initiative in the United States.

Centers for Disease Control and Prevention
1600 Clifton Road
Atlanta, GA 30333
(800) 232-4636
www.cdc.gov
The Centers for Disease Control and Prevention (CDC) provides resources and education in the area of illness, infectious diseases, and health promotion.

Cleft Palate Foundation Cleft Line
1504 East Franklin Street, Suite 102
Chapel Hill, NC 27514-2820
(919) 933-9044
www.cleftline.org
The Cleft Line provides referral to a local support group for parents of babies with facial birth defects.

DONA International
1582 S. Parker Road, Suite 201
Denver, CO 80231
(888) 788-3662
www.dona.org
DONA can help you locate a doula in your area.

Human Milk Banking Association of North America
1500 Sunday Drive, Suite 102
Raleigh, NC 27607
(919) 861-4530
www.hmbana.org
This organization provides guidance and policies regarding the collection, storage, processing, and use of human milk.

International Board of Lactation Consultant Examiners (IBLCE)
6402 Arlington Boulevard, Suite 350
Falls Church, VA 22042
(703) 560-7330
http://americas.iblce.org
IBLCE oversees the process of examination and certification of lactation consultants.

International Lactation Consultant Association (ILCA)
2501 Aerial Center Parkway, Suite 103
Morrisville, NC 27560
(888) 452-2478
(919) 861-5577
www.ilca.org
ILCA is the professional organization of lactation consultants and may
be able to provide assistance with locating a lactation consultant in
your area.

La Leche League International, Inc.
957 N. Plum Grove Road
Schaumburg, IL 60173
(847) 519-7730
(800) 525-3243
www.llli.org
La Leche League International provides a directory of volunteer personnel who coordinate the activities of local groups, as well as a comprehensive website with current information about breastfeeding, a catalog
of publications and additional breastfeeding resources, and guides to international meetings and breastfeeding seminars for health care professionals. See local phone listings to locate meetings in your area.

National Organization of Mothers of Twins Club
2000 Mallory Lane, Suite 130-600
Franklin, TN 37067-8231
(248) 231-4480
www.nomotc.org
This organization is a network of nearly five hundred clubs representing
parents of twins, triplets, and quadruplets. It fosters development of
local support groups, participates in research projects, and will put you
in touch with local chapters.

The National Women's Health Information Center
(800) 994-9662
www.womenshealth.gov
This service of the Office on Women's Health in the U.S. Department
of Health and Human Services has a program called the Business Case
for Breastfeeding. This is a comprehensive program designed to educate
employers about the value of supporting breastfeeding employees in the
workplace.

Nursing Mothers Counsel
P.O. Box 5024
San Mateo, CA 94402-0024
(650) 327-6455
www.nursingmothers.org
The Nursing Mothers Counsel provides information and publications
on breastfeeding for mothers and health care professionals.

United States Breastfeeding Committee
2025 M Street, NW, Suite 800
Washington, DC 20036-3309
(202) 367-1132
www.usbreastfeeding.org
The U.S. Breastfeeding Committee aims to support ongoing breastfeeding projects and develop a strategic plan for breastfeeding in the
United States.

United States Department of Health and Human Services
200 Independence Avenue, SW
Washington, DC 20201
877-696-6775
www.health.gov/DietaryGuidelines
The U.S. Department of Health and Human Services and the Department of Agriculture have jointly published the Dietary Guidelines for
Americans every five years since 1980. The guidelines provide authorita-

tive advice for people two years and older about how good dietary habits can promote health and reduce risk for major chronic diseases. They serve as the basis for federal food and nutrition education programs.

U.S. Lactation Consultant Association
2501 Aerial Center Parkway, Suite 103
Morrisville, NC 27560
(919) 861-4543
www.uslca.org
The United States Lactation Consultant Association is organized for the advocacy of the International Board Certified Lactation Consultant.

Wellstart International
P.O. Box 80877
San Diego, CA 92138-0877
(619) 295-5192
www.wellstart.org
Wellstart International promotes breastfeeding on a local, national, and international level by training and equipping health care professionals and developing breastfeeding curricula, materials, and policy.

WIC: Special Supplemental Nutrition Program for Women, Infants, and Children
National WIC Association
2001 S Street, NW, Suite 580
Washington, DC 20009
(202) 232-5492
www.nwica.org
www.fns.usda.gov/wic
The goals of the National Breastfeeding Promotion Campaign of WIC are to encourage participants to begin and to continue breastfeeding by increasing referrals to WIC for breastfeeding support, increasing public acceptance and support of breastfeeding, and providing support and technical assistance to WIC state and local professionals in the promo-

tion of breastfeeding. Consult local phone listings for offices in your area or call the local health department.

Books to Share with Children

I Eat at Mommy's, Anna E. Bradley-McBeth
Will There Be a Lap for Me? Dorothy Corey, Nancy Poydar
Maggie's Weaning, Mary Joan Deutschbein
About Twins, Shelly Rotner, Sheila M. Kelly
We Like to Nurse, Chia Martin, Shukyo Lin Mithuna
See How You Grow, Patricia Pearse, Edwina Riddell
Michele, the Nursing Toddler, Jane M. Pinczuk, Barbara Murray
On Mother's Lap, Ann Herbert Scott, Glo Coalson
The Best Gifts, Marsha Forchuk Skrypuch, Halina Below
The Cuddlers, Stacy Towle-Morgan, Marvin Jarboe
A Baby Just Like Me, Susan Winter
Mama's Milk/Mama Me Alimenta, Michael Elsohn Ross, Ashley Wolff
Look What I See! Where Can I Be? In the Neighborhood, Dia L Michels, Michael J. N. Bowles
If My Mom Were a Platypus: Mammal Babies and Their Mothers, Dia L. Michels, Andrew Barthelmes

Breastfeeding Record

Use this record when you breastfeed and when your baby needs a diaper change during the first week. This will help you keep track of how well your baby is breastfeeding. Look at the sample.

1. Circle the hour closest to when your baby starts each breast-feeding.
2. Circle the **W** when the baby has a wet diaper.
3. Circle the **BM** when the baby has a bowel movement.

It is okay for your baby to have more wet diapers or bowel movements than the goal. If your baby has less than the goal, call your pediatrician or lactation specialist.

SAMPLE	GOAL
①2③4 5⑥7 8⑨10⑪noon 1②3④5 6⑦8 9⑩11 12	At least 8-12
Wet Diapers Ⓦ	1
Bowel Movements—black ⓑⓜ ⓑⓜ	1

On the first day the baby fed 9 times, wet 1 diaper and had 2 dirty diapers.

BIRTHDAY	GOAL
1 2 3 4 5 6 7 8 9 10 11 noon 1 2 3 4 5 6 7 8 9 10 11 12	At least 8–12
Wet Diapers W	1
Bowel Movements—black BM	1

ONE DAY OLD	GOAL
1 2 3 4 5 6 7 8 9 10 11 noon 1 2 3 4 5 6 7 8 9 10 11 12	At least 8–12
Wet Diapers W W	2
Bowel Movements—black BM BM	2

TWO DAYS OLD	GOAL
1 2 3 4 5 6 7 8 9 10 11 noon 1 2 3 4 5 6 7 8 9 10 11 12	At least 8–12
Wet Diapers W W W	3
Bowel Movements—green BM BM	2

THREE DAYS OLD	GOAL
1 2 3 4 5 6 7 8 9 10 11 noon 1 2 3 4 5 6 7 8 9 10 11 12	At least 8–12
Wet Diapers W W W W	4
Bowel Movements—yellow-green BM BM BM	3

FOUR DAYS OLD	GOAL
1 2 3 4 5 6 7 8 9 10 11 noon 1 2 3 4 5 6 7 8 9 10 11 12	At least 8–12
Wet Diapers W W W W W	5
Bowel Movements—yellow BM BM BM	3

FIVE DAYS OLD	GOAL
1 2 3 4 5 6 7 8 9 10 11 noon 1 2 3 4 5 6 7 8 9 10 11 12	At least 8–12
Wet Diapers W W W W W W	6
Bowel Movements—yellow BM BM BM BM	4

SIX DAYS OLD	GOAL
1 2 3 4 5 6 7 8 9 10 11 noon 1 2 3 4 5 6 7 8 9 10 11 12	At least 8–12
Wet Diapers W W W W W W	6–8
Bowel Movements—yellow BM BM BM BM	4–12

DATE: _____	GOAL
1 2 3 4 5 6 7 8 9 10 11 noon 1 2 3 4 5 6 7 8 9 10 11 12	At least 8–12
Wet Diapers W W W W W W	6–8
Bowel Movements—yellow BM BM BM BM	4–12

DATE: _____	GOAL
1 2 3 4 5 6 7 8 9 10 11 noon 1 2 3 4 5 6 7 8 9 10 11 12	At least 8–12
Wet Diapers W W W W W W	6–8
Bowel Movements—yellow BM BM BM BM	4–12

DATE: _____	GOAL
1 2 3 4 5 6 7 8 9 10 11 noon 1 2 3 4 5 6 7 8 9 10 11 12	At least 8–12
Wet Diapers W W W W W W	6–8
Bowel Movements—yellow BM BM BM BM	4–12

Index